STOP
PROCRASTINATING
START
LIVING

THREE BOOKS IN ONE

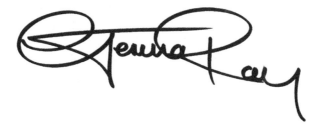

Copyright © 2021 Gemma Ray

All rights reserved. This book or any portion thereof may not be reproduced or used in any manner whatsoever without the express written permission of the publisher except for the use of brief quotations in a book review.

ISBN 9798537948605

www.gemmaray.com

This book is dedicated to YOU.

The future version of you.

That future version of you who is just a product of repeated decisions.

Let me show you how to make some positive ones so you can meet your future self.

Contents: Book 1 - Six Steps

Step 1 - Prepare to Fail & Forgive the Failure 23
Step 2 - Prepare the Right Environment 29
Step 3 - Get in the Right Frame of Mind 31
Step 4 - Use a Timer to Get Realistic and Focused With Your Productivity 34
Step 5 - Stay Accountable 38
Step 6 - Drop Perfectionism 43
In Summary 49
Space for Additional Notes and Learnings 50

Contents: Book 2 - Self Discipline

Title Page 59
Introduction 73
Setting Your Goals 76
Step 1- Establishing Your Solid Morning Routine 96
Step 2 - Make Your Health a Habit 114
Step 3 - Ways to Stay Accountable 132
Step 4 - How to Avoid Goal Overwhelm 142
Step 5 - Getting Out Of Your Own Way 150
Step 6 - Sprint vs Slow 161
Step 7 - How to Schedule Like a Boss 170
Step 9 - Rest, Relax and Reward 184
Step 10 - Failure v Success 190
Conclusion 195

Contents: Book 3: Stop Procrastinating

Title Page 201
Chapter 1 - What is Procrastination Anyway? 221
Chapter 2 - Drop the Perfectionism 228
Chapter 3 - Count Down and Take Action 236
Chapter 4 - The Two Minute Rule for Getting Things Done 242
Chapter 5 - The Five Minute Rule - More Realistic Than Two Minutes? 247
Chapter 6 - Implementation Intentions 251
Chapter 7 - Habit Stacking 258
Chapter 8 - Use the Pomodoro Method 264
Chapter 9 - Create a Tidy Space 269
Chapter 10 - Visualise Yourself Productive (Or a Success!) 273
Chapter 11 - Get in the Zone 279
Chapter 13 - Practise Forgiveness 292
Chapter 14 - List Your Fears 297
Chapter 15 - Put it in the F*ck-it Bucket and Move on 301
Chapter 16 - Write Down Your Wins 306
Chapter 17 - Create a Lightbulb List 312
Chapter 19 - Binaural Beats 323
Chapter 20 - Have a Power Nap 326
Chapter 23 - The Accountability Mirror 339

Chapter 24 - Audit Your Phone Use 343

Chapter 25 - Factor in Some Play 348

Chapter 26 - The Dopamine Fast and Digital Detox 351

Chapter 27 - Enjoy The Discomfort 357

Chapter 28 - Final Words 361

Acknowledgements 364

Appendix 366

Welcome to the Stop Procrastinating and Start Living Series

This 3-books-in-1 bumper edition contains everything you need to stop procrastinating, take action and succeed with your goals.

The first book in this series, Stop Procrastinating in Six Steps, is part mini-book and part workbook. I created this purposely knowing that many people download my books when they are feeling stuck and need to take action.

Stop Procrastinating in Six Steps has been designed to be read and the exercises completed in around an hour. This first short, sharp and simple introduction to action taking will really help you get clear on what might have been holding you back so far and how to proceed with a new plan and a fresh perspective.

Once you have completed Stop Procrastinating in Six Steps, the next book in the series is Self Discipline. This how-to guide contains 10 specific ways to instil a bit more discipline into your life. I do discipline a little differently than most because it is something I continue to struggle with on a daily basis. What really helped me and completely changed my life was reframing discipline as the highest form of self-care. I like to think of discipline as a series of promises to ourselves that we keep. When we keep our promises to ourselves we develop self-trust and when we trust ourselves to be able to do what we say we will do, we develop self-belief, It is that self-belief and strong inner knowing that "we've got this" that cements the habits loops and behaviour changes we need to achieve our goals.

Book 3 is Stop Procrastinating and Start Living. I thoroughly enjoyed researching and writing this book that is backed with hacks, hints and tips to take action when procrastination strikes. Read it from cover to cover but also use it as a tool to come back to whenever you're sitting staring into space and looking for that kick in the butt to take action. I like to flick through the pages at speed, stop on a random chapter and use the tools outlined to help me stop faffing about and get to work.

If you have any feedback on the books I'd love to hear from you. I can be contacted at gemma@gemmaray.com or you can follow me on social media:

Facebook: @gemmaraypullyourfingerout

Instagram: @gemmadeeray

Twitter: @gemmadeeray

I wish you the very best on your quest to level up your life, get inspired into action and achieve your goals.

Gem

STOP PROCRASTINATING IN SIX STEPS

Get Back on Track With Six Powerful Productivity Strategies for Success

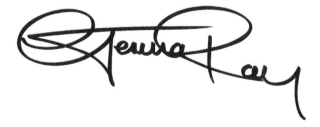

Copyright © 2021 Gemma Ray

All rights reserved. This book or any portion thereof may not be reproduced or used in any manner whatsoever without the express written permission of the publisher except for the use of brief quotations in a book review.

Other books by Gemma Ray

2018 - Self Discipline: A How-To Guide to Stop Procrastination and Achieve Your Goals in 10 Steps

2020 - Stop Procrastinating and Start Living: Beat Procrastination and Boost Productivity for Self Care and Success

www.gemmaray.com

For my friend, Leah Bramich, who moaned that she didn't have time to procrastinate by reading a full book on procrastination. You were the inspiration for writing this mini version!

More than Just a Mini Book

I know how difficult it is to make and maintain changes in your life. Discipline is really tough for many of us! I wanted to create additional tools that would help you to understand and improve your own relationship with self-discipline, so I would love to offer you a gift as a valued reader.

Special offer! FREE Online Goal setting Masterclass & Workbook
To accompany this book, I have created a powerful Goal Setting Masterclass and workbook. Designed to help you get clarity on your goals, shine a light on what's been holding you back and eradicate procrastination once and for all.

Get your free gifts at **www.gemmaray.com/bonus**

Procrastination Busting Starts Here...

Thank you for downloading this eBook which aims to help you go from procrastination panic to diligently disciplined in six steps.

I'm Gemma Ray, author of the Amazon #1 best sellers Self-Discipline, a How-to Guide to Stop Procrastination & Achieve Your Goals and Stop Procrastinating and Start Living. I have successfully learned how to overcome procrastination and developed self-discipline in my life and the lives of others.

I'm not someone who is ex-military or likes to do discipline with aggression. I teach discipline and procrastination busting methods to real people with real jobs, real families, real commitments and real lives. I believe there is no such thing as being lazy. Research suggests we procrastinate because one or more of our basic needs are not being met. I have created this mini book as the perfect thing for you to procrastinate on! This isn't as long as my published books, is easy to read in one sitting and contains easy to action hints, tips and hacks you can put into practice straight away. It is the foolproof system of pressing an imaginary panic button when procrastination teeters on the verge of endangering your discipline.

Procrastination has the power to destroy your mood, add to your stress, make you feel like a failure and get you into trouble.

A better, brighter you can emerge on the other side of overwhelm and these foolproof strategies could be the key to achieving your goals.

Need some extra help? Check out **www.gemmaray.com** for more productivity resources.

Step 1

Prepare to Fail & Forgive the Failure

Yes, that's right, I said prepare to fail. If you're reading this eBook the chances are you're someone who is already struggling with procrastination. It affects all of us! Even that super-human colleague of yours or that focused friend who always seems to have their life together.

So what do I mean by preparing to fail? Well, first of all we start with something really important.

FORGIVENESS

Scientific studies have proven that procrastination is linked to feelings of shame. When we start to work on our procrastination tendencies, we should start with forgiveness of the self. It does not matter what has happened in the past, you cannot change what has already happened. You only have today onwards. So draw a line under what has happened in the past with procrastination and get ready to move on. If you'd like to read up on this further, look up the Carlton University study titled *I Forgive Myself, Now I Can Study: How self-forgiveness for procrastinating can reduce future procrastination*.

I want to help you through a process of self-forgiveness through the following journal prompts. Writing things down helps you to process your thoughts. If you are not a fan of journaling, you could use these prompts as a talking point with a trusted friend, relative or coworker.

Write down the tasks that you tend to procrastinate on the most. Think about the things you put off that cause you the most stress.

Thinking about those tasks you procrastinate on the most, how can you forgive yourself for not always getting them done?

Now complete this sentence:

I forgive myself for _____ *[task you procrastinate on]* I cannot change what has happened in the past, but I can look to the future which is within my control.

Please take a moment to really feel into that self-forgiveness. It is very important to let go of what has been and that you cannot change. Allowing yourself a moment of self-forgiveness will help you start with a fresh new perspective.

The second part of this first tip is to:

PREPARE TO FAIL

That's right! You need to set up a strategy for the NEXT time you get caught out by the pain of procrastination.

Have you ever trained in First Aid? The art of administering CPR or treating a burn or dealing with a fracture is covered in a course so you know what to do in the event of an emergency.

This comparison is a little dramatic but I want you to think about creating a First Aid strategy for the next time procrastination hits.

The first thing to do is identify the signs you're about to enter a procrastination wormhole. Procrastination is often our response to stress, fear, overwhelm and is NOT necessarily laziness.

Many people get angry with themselves when procrastination strikes. They feel like they've let themselves down. They feel like they've failed. They feel like they can't trust themselves.

These are all normal emotional responses to the effects and consequences of procrastination. So in order to undo this emotional response to overwhelm and stress, we need to be prepared for how procrastination starts in the first place.

So let's get to know you and your behaviours a little better in this eBook. Use a notepad or journal to answer some of the exercises.

What Do You Procrastinate on Most and Why Is It Important?

Are there specific tasks in your life that you always struggle to feel motivated to do?

Taking the list you have written from question 1, I want you to identify three main tasks that you always seem to put off. We are going to examine why each one is important. What does it mean if you get these tasks done? More money, more organised? Less stress down the line? Someone else's happiness?

You might want to use this format:

I procrastinate on (task #1)

Getting task #1 completed is important to me because:

I procrastinate on (task #2)

Getting task #2 completed is important to me because:

I procrastinate on (task #3)

Getting task #3 completed is important to me because:

Identify Your Procrastination Warning Signs

Outline key things you 'do' 'say' or 'think' when you can feel the prickle of procrastination about to take over you.

It might be that you comfort eat. You might think it wise to suddenly start binge watching a Netflix series. You might bury yourself in your phone.

Have a really good think about your own patterns.

When you're really avoiding tasks, what do you tend to do instead?

_____
_____
_____

What patterns of behaviour do you present?

_____
_____
_____

Are there any patterns to you acting like this?

_____
_____
_____

What distracts you?

_____
_____
_____

What do you need to do less of in these scenarios?

What usually gets you motivated to start? (Or do you panic at the last moment?)

Keep these behaviours that you have outlined in mind. We will revisit them later in this eBook.

Step 2

Prepare the Right Environment

Your environment is everything! Getting in the right environment free of distractions that can derail you makes tasks much easier.

If you work in an open plan office then it's likely you will be distracted by colleagues many times throughout the day.

- Could you book a private meeting room to help you focus?
- If you work from home, where do you work from?
- Do you have a dedicated space? Is it clean and tidy?
- Does it light you up and make you feel good?

I know tidying a desk is a common example of procrastination but there's scientific research about the need for things to be in order before you can focus. So if you need to tidy your desk, get it done but set a strict timer.

Environment Exercise

I want you to think about something you procrastinate on a regular basis or a task that is pressing that you can't seem to get started or motivated to do. Something that you just always put off starting or doing.

What is your environment like when you're trying to attempt this task? Describe it, or even better go to that place now when answering these questions.

What are the positives in this environment?

What are the negatives? Who or what distracts you?

Now think about being more productive in this particular environment, what would create the optimum condition here to complete this task?

(Describe it in as much detail as possible - how are you going to work best?)

Have a good think about your environment around those irritating tasks you put off. There will usually be a way you can make the environment work better for you and put you in the right frame of mind to tackle your tasks. Which leads nicely onto...

Step 3

Get in the Right Frame of Mind

Are you mentally prepped and ready to kick procrastination's butt?

If you're in a state of stress, upset, discomfort or overwhelm it is time to regain some mental toughness and get your mind prepared to win.

Deep Breathing Techniques

If you've been feeling overwhelmed and stressed out, working on your breathing can be a great starting point.

There are many meditation tracks on YouTube that can help you get in the zone with your breathing techniques. You may have also heard of Wim Hof? If not, Google him and his specialist breathing techniques that many people swear by to set them up for the day. He has an app called WHM that is really good.

Music Anchoring

Have you ever seen the beginning of a boxing match? What do the fighters do? They come into the ring to a specific predetermined piece of music, that means something to them. It's the music that gets them fired up and ready in their winning mentality.

Music has a great power to change our conscious emotive state. There will be songs in your life that instantly take you back to a moment in time, a memory or a person. If you don't already have a piece of music think of a song that is going to be YOUR anti-procrastination track. It's going to be your song that you come into the ring with and knock out procrastination in one punch.

You could use this track on your way to work in the car, on your way to the gym, on your running playlist or even just play it at your desk through your headphones when you're about to start that important piece of work.

What is your ultimate favourite feelgood track that could get you in the zone?

Bonus exercise: if you have more than one track that uplifts you and makes you feel motivated then why not create a digital playlist on your streaming service of choice. Create your GSD (Get Stuff Done) playlist to help you get in the mood, the frame of mind and motivate you into action.

The Five Second Rule

International speaker and best selling author Mel Robbins became famous using her 5 Second Rule technique. It's pretty simple, and the idea was inspired by a rocket launch she watched on TV.

5…4…3…2…1…lift off!

Mel realised that her own procrastination could be overcome using this same technique. 5,4,3,2,1 and action! Getting yourself in the right frame of mind might include the 5 second rule before you start work. 5…4…3…2…1 - START! It could be your mental mantra to get you out of procrastination and into being productive.

Switch Off and Remove Distractions

Did you know? It takes around 23 minutes once distracted to go back to a task. So every time a notification pops up on your phone or a coworker interrupts you at your desk or that email pings into your inbox, what happens? You get distracted. And then it's 23 minutes to get back in the zone. Is it any wonder we all procrastinate?!

Headphones are a great way to switch off, whether you choose to play any music out of them or not! Wearing headphones in work instantly tells your colleagues you're working and focused and don't want to be distracted.

Personally, I can't have too much music in the background while I am working. Anything with words and a vocal distracts me so I tend to listen to classical music while writing or I do use binaural beats which I highly recommend. Binaural beats are sound waves played at specific frequencies. The frequencies are meant to enhance the tasks you are doing such as writing, resting, problem solving. Type 'binaural beats' into your app store of choice and have a play with the apps out there. I highly recommend a Binaural Beat soundtrack or audio programme for focused work.

Remove distractions if you need to focus, including:

- Turn your phone off
- If you can't turn your phone off, turn off your phone notifications temporarily
- Switch off your email programme
- Turn off your office phone
- Book out a meeting room or quiet space if you have noisy colleagues
- Ask to work from home if this environment works for you

Is there anything else you could do to get in the right frame of mind? Make a note of it here:

_____

_____

_____

_____

Step 4

Use a Timer to Get Realistic and Focused With Your Productivity

Do you actually know the average time your most procrastinated-on tasks take you? I bet you'd be shocked! This is a great exercise you can do today to help the next time you find yourself procrastinating. I advise this exercise for everyone who finds themselves putting things off.

Start to time everything in your life. Do it over the course of a couple of days or a week and make a list. I get my clients to do this and it completely changes the way they work. It is the one thing that helps time management, organising your diary and overcoming procrastination when it feels like overwhelm.

Time everyday tasks in your life and business. Prioritise auditing the tasks you tend to procrastinate on the most. The very first time I did this exercise and when I get clients to do this, I advise the following:

- Set the digital timer going on your phone
- Turn the phone over so the screen faces down (and doesn't distract you)
- Work as your usual speed on the different tasks you are tracking

When I first did this exercise I was working full-time as a done-for-you copywriter. I was procrastinating on a lot of client work which meant I would then panic, do it all late at night, not rest properly and always feel like I was chasing my tail and doing a crap job. I'd sometimes look at my schedule and wonder how the heck I could fit all my work in, causing overwhelm, Yet I'd find myself on my phone instead of working just making the problem a lot worse.

I realised that the average long form social media post takes me 8 minutes to write. So when a client wants me to write 30 posts I know that I need 4 hours to complete this. I worked out that the average 3 minute client video takes 5 hours to edit. It takes me 45 minutes to write a newsletter and depending on the length of the award entry, it takes around 6 hours to complete an award application.

Once I had these lists and lists of times that tasks take me, it helped me be more realistic in planning my time. Rather than looking at my watch thinking "I don't have time to write this right now" and overthink it, I could be realistic and think "Yes, I've got an hour let's see if I can get it done." Because attempting SOMETHING was better than not getting started at all.

When I timed my regular work tasks it really did change my life. It became a game. Me against the clock and I was able to get realistic with my workload. I was able to work smarter and more efficiently but I was also able to say no to things that I knew I didn't have time for.

I'd urge you to do the same and time all those tasks you procrastinate on.

Do this with as many tasks as you can that you tend to put off and have a more realistic picture of how long things take. You won't feel as overwhelmed next time you look at that long to-do list.

You'll be in a position where you can really plan your tasks ahead with the time you have available and you'll also feel more empowered to say a firm "no" to those things you know you won't have time for.

My main recurring tasks at work are:	**Time**

My main recurring tasks at home are: *Time*

....

....

....

....

The Pomodoro Technique

There's another way to use a timer that will help you feel more focused, productive and help stop overwhelm when you're working.

Did your grandma or anyone in the family ever have a mechanical kitchen timer?? Well if you've seen these before, chances are you've used them for timing boiled eggs or that chicken in the oven. I love to use one of these tomato timers for a productive way of working called The Pomodoro Technique.

Francesco Cirillo found that in his college years he wasn't using his study time well and would get distracted. So he grabbed his tomato shaped kitchen timer and developed the Pomodoro Technique which has now been adopted by millions of people looking to focus and knuckle down on their tasks.

The Pomodoro Technique involves breaking down tasks into 25 minute chunks of time. The idea is that you work for 25 focused minutes on ONE TASK and that one task only, and then take a 5 minute break.

After four consecutive working time blocks, you take a longer break, around 20 or 30 minutes.

Pomodoro 1	10:00	Write blog
Break	10:25	Make a coffee
Pomodoro 2	10:30	Format blog and post it
Break	10:55	Check social media

I also recommend having this tomato timer or grabbing an inexpensive mechanical timer so you always have it to hand. Yes, you can use digital options or the timer on your phone, but I found these far too easy to override. A mechanical timer was one of the best things I ever invested in to keep me on track and focused in my work.

I have a free Pomodoro PDF tracker you can download and use if you'd like to try this method.

Go to **gemmaray.com/pomodoro** to get your free digital Pomodoro planner.

Step 5

Stay Accountable

Have you ever had a partner on something to do with work or training? Maybe you've had a gym buddy or diet buddy in the past? Perhaps you've had a proper accountability buddy or a coach?

Staying accountable really helps you to eradicate procrastination. Depending on your accountability style, most people benefit from having someone to check in with and remain accountable to.

According to a study by the Association for Talent Development, you're 95% more likely to stick to a goal if you have someone to stay accountable to.

Ways to Stay Accountable

If you struggle with procrastination in particular, then accountability around getting started on tasks is usually a positive exercise.

Get an Accountability Buddy

Is there someone who you can check in with regularly, whether that is a professional coach or mentor who you pay, or simply a friend or colleague? This person needs to be someone you trust and most definitely someone who will not trigger you. You need to think of someone who will be very supportive.

Agree on a set of actions with your accountability buddy and check-in at regular intervals on the tasks you achieve, as you tick them off your to-do list. If you haven't achieved them, be honest and work together on being more realistic in your actions to get your tasks completed.

You could also hire a professional accountability mentor (like me!) who will have systematic methods and processes to help you stick to your weekly actions.

Who could you connect with to help you stay accountable?

_____

_____

_____

Start a Blog

When I speak of starting a 'blog', this doesn't necessarily have to be on a blogging platform. A lot of people might get scared of the prospect of sorting out the tech and investment needed for a blogging website. Instead, people keep it simple and inexpensive by starting their 'blog' on social media. I know that technically this isn't a proper blog in the traditional sense, but just getting down your thoughts and feelings as you move through your journey can be beneficial. It doesn't matter which platform you choose, putting your action steps out there to the world and using your writing on social media or a blogging platform can keep you accountable. Plenty of people start dedicated Instagram profiles or just post on their social media to stay accountable. If you wanted to start your own proper blog with your own website, that is a possibility too. Just remember the time it will take to keep it going. You don't want to add another task into the mix if you are already overwhelmed!

One of the simplest ways to stay accountable using social media is to post your daily actions and then report back on them. At the time of writing, I have been doing this myself for around six months now, and I love my daily 'Ta Dah' lists on my Instagram stories. You can follow me here **www.instagram.com/gemmadeeray**, and you'll see the daily lists I post. If you'd like a copy of the Instagram story templates to use yourself, you can download them for free here: **www.gemmaray.com/instatemplates**. I would love for you to tag me into your stories so I can see what you're getting up to.

Start a WhatsApp or Facebook Group

If you're on a mission and working towards a sporting endeavour or weight loss, why not round up a few like-minded friends and create a dedicated group where you all keep one another accountable?

You can post your daily progress in the group and help inspire each other on. I am part of a running group, and there is nothing more motivating than a sea of Strava maps and run times to make you want to lace up your trainers. I also have a group with friends who are on a fitness mission and their recipes and healthy food inspiration on WhatsApp are very inspirational and gives me lots of ideas for new recipes.

Hire a Coach

If you really need the help and dedicated support, consider hiring a coach. If you are struggling with procrastination in your day to day work, you may want to look into a business coach or mentor. If it is your health and fitness that is the priority you just can't seem to prioritise then consider hiring a nutritionist, personal trainer or online well-being coach.

There are coaches for every sector and challenge that you may have. I work as an accountability mentor and a communications coach. I love to help people stick to their action steps to achieve their goals, and I adore helping business owners to get clear with their communications so they can market and grow their business.

Join a Group

There are so many groups on social media platforms like Facebook and LinkedIn that could help keep you accountable. Whether it's fitness, business or even more niche subjects related to your hobbies, if you search for it, there will be a group on it!

You might also wish to join a group in person, like a running or sporting group. The community element of the group acts as brilliant accountability to keep you wanting to return and participate in more events.

After reading this chapter, spend a few minutes outlining ways in which you could be accountable to achieve your goals. Think about the people you could ask for help or the groups you could join. What or who could help you achieve your goals quicker?

Step 6

Drop Perfectionism

Ahhh perfectionism is an absolute nightmare, isn't it? Most of us perfectionists don't even admit we are a perfectionist. If you've ever waited for the right moment, if you've ever worried about other people's criticism of your actions or if you've always been afraid of making mistakes then chances are you're a perfectionist.

Research suggests that perfectionism can be closely related to depression and self-esteem. It makes sense if you think about it. If we believe negative things about ourselves and we tell ourselves that we aren't good enough, then we will struggle to accept that our actions and the work or outcomes we produce are good enough.

But who decides what is actually good enough? Surely doing SOMETHING and it not being absolutely perfect is better than doing nothing at all?

There are a few different types of perfectionists, but we usually fall into these common categories:

- The "I'll do it soon" perfectionist. This is the one that never starts. The one who desperately wants to achieve something but immediately starts doubting themselves and thinks they can't do it. They don't even start, and they don't even try.
- The "My standards are too high" perfectionist. This perfectionist makes a start, sets

a goal but sets the goal so high that they always fail. They work hard, sometimes too hard, but never seem to appreciate what they have achieved or celebrate their successes. This person might also want everything to be perfect before they take action. They think they need to exercise every day to lose weight, set a goal to write an unrealistic number of words to get the book finished or set impossible run distances to tackle in a month.

I used those examples above because they are my previous examples and where I failed. If things were not perfect, I would throw the towel in too quickly.

Personally, I've found that stripping goals back into the tiniest of actions is the way to overcome perfectionism. When I think too far in advance of the big goal and what I want to achieve, I immediately think I'm not good enough, and I'm paralysed by procrastination.

In his book Atomic Habits, James Clear states that every new habit should start with a two-minute action. This is about mastering the habit of showing up, not about doing things perfectly.

He states that you can break down any major goal into one simple, straightforward action that should not take more than two minutes. For example, "Run three miles" becomes "Tie my running shoes" or one that I have found really useful is stop saying "Write 2,000 words" and instead say "Open my manuscript". If you start with the smallest action, complete it, get used to winning and master how it feels, you will naturally start to add more to your actions.

- So running a marathon is **extremely hard**
- Running a 5k is **hard**
- Walking 10,000 steps daily is **moderately difficult**
- Walking 10 minutes is **easy**
- Tying your running shoes is **very easy**

Using my example of writing a book, you could use the scale above

- Launching a best-selling book is **extremely hard**
- Editing a book is **hard**
- Writing a book is moderately **difficult**

- Writing a chapter is **easy**
- Opening your manuscript is **very easy**

Could you use the same scale for anything you regularly procrastinate on?

What new habits do you want to form that you could start off with only a two-minute action or decide on an action step with significantly less expectation than achieving your goal in one session?

Learn to Surrender

Dropping perfectionism also requires a sense of surrender. You really have to let go of that need for everything to be perfect.

- There will never be a perfect time
- There will never be perfect circumstances
- Anything you produce will never be 100% perfect

To overcome perfectionism, focus on getting things DONE, not getting things perfect. So using all the strategies outlined in this book, could you just work on getting things done?

Could you set a timer to see how long things take to get done and once done, accept they are done? (No tweaking, changing and fiddling later).

Could you use the Pomodoro timer to break your tasks into 25 minutes of focused action and see how you get on?

Could you accept that the environment you are in will never be perfect so instead work on making it as best as it can be? Remember - remove distractions, get that winning song on, get fired up!

But, above all can you truly accept that things will never ever be 100% perfect? When you focus on done over perfect, when you are regularly getting things done, over and over again, you will eventually feel empowered to tackle your tasks with ease. There is a wonderful phrase I want you to write on your mirrors, on post-it notes in the car or your desk, on every journal or notebook:

"I am enough."

Remind yourself of this every time you feel the paralysing effects of perfectionism and try with all of your might to just take that first step. A blank document cannot be edited. You cannot run a marathon without taking that first step. Your book will not write itself. You ARE enough, and your efforts are enough. So take action and see where your action steps take you.

After reading this chapter, think about your relationship with perfectionism.

What goals have you put on hold or been stuck with perfectionism procrastination paralysis because things aren't 'perfect'?

Where have you been getting overwhelmed thinking your goals are too big and scary, so you've not taken any action?

Where can you cut yourself some slack and take your goals back to basics?

What are the smallest and tiniest action steps you can commit to that will get you moving towards achieving your biggest and most important goals?

In Summary

It's really easy for me to say "Just try these action steps!" to stop procrastinating. When you're in that mindset, it is super difficult to break! Pushing the procrastination panic button requires you to create some forward-thinking strategies.

When you know the signs of your own procrastination, and when you've developed a strategy to combat it, it gets easier to overcome each time.

That's why I believe learning about yourself, asking yourself questions about your own fears and exploring why things are important to you is the key to start to train your brain to reduce your procrastination time gradually.

If you really are struggling with procrastination, then I have a number of free downloads available via my website at **www.gemmaray.com** You may also choose to join my FREE Level:Up Facebook community where we support one another with all aspects of productivity and goal achievement to level up in all areas of our lives. To join the group, please click here at **bit.do/levelupfacebookgroup**. Don't forget to answer the questions and agree to the rules first.

90 Day Accountability Programme – Change Your Life One Decision at a Time!

If you know you need a little more support to get inspired into action, I run a paid 90-day programme three times per year. Entry to the group is by application only to ensure you are the right fit for the group. We operate as a tight-knit structured and focused group of people who all help to achieve goals and support one another. To apply for the next 90-day programme, please email gemma@gemmaray.com to find out the latest dates and availability.

Space for Additional Notes and Learnings

Stop Procrastinating in Six Steps

About Gemma Ray

Gemma Ray should have a PhD in procrastination. Her book on self-discipline (that she had no self-discipline to write) continues to top the bestseller charts.

Her second book Stop Procrastinating and Start Living was a runaway success gaining bestseller status and the #1 spot in over 20 categories in UK and US Amazon bookstores.

Gemma writes from the heart for real people who need a hand pulling their finger out to take action and level up all areas of their life. She has written for a number of publications, newspapers, blogs and businesses before realising a childhood dream of becoming an author. She writes "the books I need to read myself" and packages her research in a personal, fun account that is easy to read and even easier to implement.

Self-proclaiming to "Not always having all my s*** together", Gemma's down-to-earth delivery and style makes you feel like you have a friend between the pages giving you simple advice over a coffee. She continues that support for her readers through her 1:1 private accountability mentoring, online coaching courses and social media channels, giving readers direct access to her no-nonsense witty retorts that makes accountability a whole lot of fun.

Gemma is a radio presenter, best selling author, content marketing and PR specialist and always the most filthy person in a WhatsApp group chat. She should probably establish the first chapter of Oversharers Anonymous, is the world's worst cook and the clumsiest person you'll ever meet.

Catch Gemma co-hosting both the Honest to Gob podcast and Body Smart podcast. Search your favourite podcast platform.

Follow her on Instagram **@gemmadeeray**

facebook.com/GemmaRayPullYourfingerOut

SELF DISCIPLINE

A How-To Guide to Stop Procrastination and Achieve Your Goals in 10 Steps

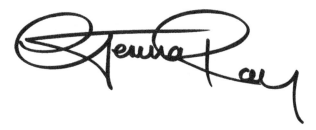

Including bonus online companion Goal Setting Masterclass to get clarity on your goals, master self-discipline and build daily habits

Copyright © 2018 Gemma Ray

Updated 2020 Gemma Ray

All rights reserved. This book or any portion thereof may not be reproduced or used in any manner whatsoever without the express written permission of the publisher except for the use of brief quotations in a book review.

www.gemmaray.com

With the most grateful heart, I dedicate this book to Ben Jones, the greatest accountability buddy the world has ever known, who became my closest ally from the other side of the globe.

Praise for Self-Discipline

"Written in Gemma's inimitable style, and littered with her quirky wit and straightforward, no-nonsense delivery, this book is best understood as a highly engaging toolkit. Packed with both step-by-step advice and a framework to build your own, personalized solution, this little gem can help you slowly, but effectively, finally beat procrastination and overwhelm. Thoroughly recommended." - Dino Tartaglia, Success Engineers

"I like the fact that the author isn't perfect and in-your-face making you feel bad. Self discipline is really hard but there are plenty of easy actions you can take from this book. A good easy read." - Pauline C, via Amazon UK

"A great book that those starting a new business, in a business or wanting to just change their mindset should read. It's so straightforward in its approach you can't put it down and instantly gives you a can do attitude." - Kelly Lou, via Amazon UK

"Since January I am down 19 pounds, killed $5500 in debt, and more organized than ever. I track my progress on my Facebook page and am inspiring so many friends, giving credit to Gemma and her easy to follow plan to get your act together." - Katie Marie, via Audible

"Perfect book for someone who struggles with discipline and organization like I did before reading this book, This was the 3rd self discipline book I've read and by far the best. Gemma has made the book as straightforward as possible and if you really give her practices a go it will change your life for the better. Enjoy:)" - Stephen, via Amazon

More than Just a Book

I know how difficult it is to make and maintain changes in your life. Discipline is really tough for many of us! (Me included). I wanted to create additional tools that would help you to understand and improve your own relationship with self-discipline, so I would love to offer you a gift as a valued reader.

FREE Online Goal setting Masterclass & Workbook

To accompany this book, I have created a powerful Goal Setting Masterclass and workbook. Designed to help you get clarity on your goals, shine a light on what's been holding you back and eradicate procrastination once and for all.

Get your free gifts at: **www.gemmaray.com/bonus**.

Prologue

"One of the most important keys to success is having the discipline to do what you know you should do, even when you don't feel like doing it."

- Unknown

A note to the reader.

Hi, I'm Gemma Ray, and I approach discipline a little bit differently from others.

I'm not ex-military, I don't run ultra-marathons, and I haven't climbed Everest. I'm a mum, a wife, a business owner and an author. I manage to fit a lot into the time I have each week, and I mentor others with kindness and compassion - rather than a boot camp shouty style experience.

I have struggled with discipline throughout my life for as long as I can remember. Many people who I mentor feel precisely the same. I help others to understand the joy of achievement through my books, online masterclasses, group programmes and free resources. I reframe discipline as an act of self-compassion. I encourage people to think about helping their future self by keeping their promises today. I plead with people to reframe discipline as something that is not about hardcore exercise, miserable restriction or doing things you don't want to do. I encourage everyone to experience a mindset shift and think of discipline as the highest form of self-care.

I believe we are all a culmination of the daily decisions that we choose to make. We are a product of our repeated decisions. For it is our daily decisions that drive action.

For example, let's say you want to lose weight (one of the most common goals). Let's say you set yourself a time limit of 90 days. Let's say you're someone who eats three meals per day. The simple maths states that the future version of you, 90 days from now, that version of you is a product of 270 meal decisions. Whatever diet or method you choose to follow, as long as you eat in a calorie deficit for those 90 days, you'll lose weight. 270 decisions at a time.

Let's pretend you want to increase the sales in your business. Right now, you know you have a conversion rate of 10 per cent on your sales calls. You want to make ten sales every week. The maths states that you will need to make an average of 100 sales calls each week to achieve this goal. You get to make the decision to make 20 sales calls per day to achieve your goal each week.

Then on the flip side of this, if you were to decide to overeat each day, indulge in excessive junk food, spend too much money every day, smoke each day, sleep every little each night (the list of bad habits could go on), over time your repeated decisions would shape the future version of yourself. How do you think that future version of a person engaging in these types of daily choices would feel, look and think?

Your daily choices and decisions will shape who you can become or the outcome of your various goals.

When I originally wrote the first version of this book, I felt continuously stuck in procrastination mode. So this book started out as a test. A test to see if I could actually research the content, write a book, publish and launch a book. The biggest test would be that people would read the book, be inspired and take action from it - resulting in them achieving their goals.

I talk about it a lot in the speeches I give on discipline and procrastination, but this is the book on self-discipline that, at first, I had no self-discipline to write. It stayed as an idea in my head until I applied everything I already knew, used a considerable amount of accountability in the form of my business partner's unwavering support, got my head down, immersed myself in research and used these techniques in the book to get this book launched and released!

In 2018, when I launched this book, I had no idea how much of a success it would become. It still continues to surprise and delight me on a daily basis. I am in awe at how many people take immediate action and start to feel better in themselves, start to trust themselves more and start to believe in their abilities.

This Book Is Not for Everyone

I don't write like many other people who publish books about self-discipline. I haven't been in the Armed Forces and undergone relentless discipline. I haven't been an Olympic athlete, and I don't have a rags-to-riches story that involved me slaving away on a business idea for years.

What I do have is an easy-to-read and even easier to implement 10 step book that has been written for the regular person who has multiple demands on their time, their brain space and their stress levels.

I write for the parents who are overcoming mum or dad guilt because they can't seem to fit in quality time with their kids.

I write for the student who knows they need to knuckle down on their studies, but no matter how hard they try, they remain stuck.

I write for the person who can't seem to get *out* of the day-to-day running of their business to work *on* their small business. They're constantly stuck in the quagmire of daily tasks and responsibilities and need a bigger picture overview of where their business is going and why.

I write for the person who has been stuck losing weight for years. I am not a dietician or a personal trainer, but I've specialised in working in the health, fitness and mindset sector for most of my career and I can tell you that dieting success is not just down to what you eat. Sustaining a successful diet phase for a long period of time will be determined by how you think more than what you consume.

I write for people who are sick of letting themselves down. Those who say "Diet starts Monday" or "I just haven't got time" or "I need to get in gear." I help people to get clear on what they want to achieve and why they want to achieve it. Then, beyond the pages of my books, I offer support in the form of free masterclasses, free resources and access to my Facebook community. Because while you might get inspired by the contents of a book, you can really benefit from ongoing and additional support to help you achieve your goals.

Self-discipline is not easy. To be fully truthful, it is still an ongoing work in progress for me. But that is OK. It gets easier the more you work on it. Just like you need to go to the gym regularly to keep your muscle tone, or eat well to keep your weight down, I believe that self-discipline and self-development are like the gym for the mind. You have to commit to it every day. The more you do, the easier it gets.

I will never profess to have all my stuff together in my head and my life. I own my own business, and I love to work hard. I balance this with being a mum and support my husband, who has a demanding job he loves. Like you, I'm busy. Really busy. But I make sure that I make time for self-disciplined actions. Although these days you'll see me reframing these actions as necessary self-care or forms of promises to myself that I choose to keep because I know that when I keep my promises to myself, I develop self-trust and that is at the heart of everything.

I am absolutely thrilled that you have purchased this book and given yourself a little time to learn more about how to flex that self-discipline muscle, develop self-trust, carve out some additional time in your life and create even more energy to achieve your goals.

I know that self-discipline doesn't start and end with reading a book, so I created some additional bonuses that I know will help you on this journey.

Bonus #1 - Goal Setting Masterclass and Companion Workbook
I have seen first-hand the power of online learning when it comes to self-development, and I wanted to create something for you, my reader, which will assist you in creating profound change and inspire you into action.

I want you to establish winning habits, positive traits and build unbreakable self-discipline to create unshakeable self-trust.

I have therefore created a Goal Setting Masterclass and accompanying workbook that will really help you to understand what you want to achieve, why you want to achieve it and then be able to confidently outline the action steps you can take to achieve your goals.

Simply visit **www.gemmaray.com/bonus** to get instant access to the masterclass and workbook.

Bonus #2 – 60 Minute Procrastination Busting Guided Focus Audio
In Step 7 – How to Schedule Like a Boss, I talk about breaking up your tasks into timed manageable chunks. This is also sometimes known as The Pomodoro Technique. Now I LOVE the Pomodoro hack. You break down your tasks into 25-minute segments (or Pomodoros)

and work on one single thing for those 25 minutes. When that Pomodoro is up, you have a 5-minute break. Once the break is over, you start on Pomodoro 2 etc.

I've used this hack for years for work, doing the chores, reading, researching, and it does work, but it's very easy to get distracted. I'm someone who can't really work with music in the background, so I tend to have relaxation music or binaural beats as my soundtrack.

I had a brainwave to create my own guided Pomodoro track. It's my 60-minute procrastination busting guided focus track, and it works!

For buying or downloading the book. You can get a copy of your FREE 60 Minute Guided Focus Audio by going to: **www.gemmaray.com/pomodoro**.

For further reading, publications and additional resources, please visit **www.gemmaray.com**.

Gemma Ray

Instagram: @gemmadeeray
Twitter: @gemmadeeray
Facebook: @GemmaRayPullYourFingerOut

Part 1

Setting Your Goals and Getting Clear on What You Want

Introduction

Self-discipline

ˌsɛlfˈdɪsəplɪn/

noun

the ability to control one's feelings and overcome one's weaknesses.
"His observance of his diet was a show of tremendous willpower and self-discipline."

Self-discipline. What is it exactly, and why is it so important?

Self-discipline is having the get-up and go to complete daily positive actions in your life that lead to inner happiness, feelings of being in control and feeling content.

You've come across this book to learn more about self-discipline, which makes me hazard a guess that you might have felt like you're struggling in this area.

I'd like to reassure you that you DO have the capability to exercise self-discipline. Everyone does. Self-discipline is the reason we get up, get washed, brush our teeth and head to work. Every one of us has the ability to use self-discipline. This book is about learning how to adopt more of it into your life.

I believe that self-discipline is three-tiered:

Habit

Motivation

Conscious Disciplined Action

Conscious Disciplined Action

When you take conscious disciplined action, you are making the necessary steps in order to achieve your goals and feel in control of your weaknesses. These actions are the foundation stones and repeated actions over time, that leads to great things. At first, it doesn't feel easy. You have to perform these action steps in a way where you're very conscious that they need to be completed, and it can feel painful and a challenge at first.

Motivation

It is possible for conscious disciplined actions to change from something forced to something you love to do, and therefore you're motivated to do it. Think about someone starting out on a health kick and going to the gym. The first few gym visits might take a lot of self-discipline to get there. Yet, soon you notice the positive effects on your body and mind and you find you WANT to go. You're motivated to head to the gym to train.

Once you've repeated enough of these daily actions, you're naturally motivated to continue the positive effects of the conscious self-discipline action steps and the process feels less forced.

Habit

Eventually, if you repeat your conscious disciplined actions habitually you find they slide into your life and daily routine with ease. Once performed consistently, these disciplined actions become so ingrained into your life that they become a habit.

No One-Size-Fits-All Model

The following chapters contain a lot of information and a lot of strategies when it comes to mastering self-discipline. Some will contradict one another. That's not me being a hypocrite. In researching and adopting many different self-discipline methods it has become evident that there is no one-size-fits-all model. You need to take what you need from this book. Be inspired, try things out, be realistic and know what would work for you and your individual personality.

I encourage you to be totally honest with yourself, accept responsibility for the choices you have made so far in your life, forgive yourself if you need to. Make notes. Scribble in the margins, add annotations on your Kindle or tablet, get a journal and make notes as you go. Or don't. That's cool too. Just say you'll try some of these techniques, because I promise when you do, you will feel like you've got your life together that little bit better.

Setting Your Goals

Goal
gəʊl/

noun
plural noun: goals
the object of a person's ambition or effort; an aim or desired result.

Have you picked up this book with a specific goal in mind already, or are you not sure what it is you're looking to accomplish?

If you aren't sure on your goal specifics, you can download the Goal Setting Masterclass and workbook that is free with this book or simply try this exercise out for size.

You will need pieces of paper, a simple list on your phone or tablet or if you're a visual person, you might want to use post-it notes.

The 100 List

Set aside some quiet time, ideally with no distractions and compile a list of 100 things you want to see, do, achieve or experience.

Your workbook as part of the Goal Setting Masterclass contains the necessary format to complete this. If you haven't already done so, you can get instant access here:

www.gemmaray.com/bonus.

The pre-work workbook sheet has a done-for-you structure for you to complete this assignment.

The first step is to write down your 100 goals which can be anything you desire. You aren't going to focus on all of them at the same time; you're just using this exercise to get clear on the things you're striving for right now at this point in your life. Don't be scared to think big and aim high. Also, don't forget about the small stuff too.

Important Note!

Now 100 seems a lot, I know. I have had feedback on this part of the book and quite a few readers found the task of writing 100 things to be a challenge. If we don't know what we want in life, how can we strive for it? And I want you to want everything - the big stuff and the small stuff. However, if it seems overwhelming, instead of setting an expectation of writing 100 things, set a timer for a specific amount of time (say 30 minutes) and write as many things as you can in the time available. This doesn't need to be perfect and there are no rules here. This is a self-motivated exercise and if you can't do 100 things, don't feel bad about it, just write what you can.

When writing your list think of different aspects of your life, work, hobbies, interests, home and relationships. Maybe there are places you want to see, health improvements you want to make or material things you want to buy. Perhaps you want to set up your own business, lose an amount of weight, reach a financial goal, build your own home, or maybe you just want to do something small like learn to cook, dine at a particular restaurant or improve your sleep.

Once you have your 100 list, go back through and categorise your wishes and goals into sections.

Are they to do with money, work, knowledge, adventure, health, family, hobbies, materialistic, etc.? Give them a colour code or a symbol so you can see at a glance which category your goals fall into. Create your own categories specific to you if you need to.

Have a look at which goals fall into which category. Is there a category that has more than others? Why do you think this is?

Assess your 100 list and pick out a top 10 that are the most important to you.

Then, when you've categorised them and picked your top 10, place them into time-specific boxes.

Which of these things on your final list of 10 things can you achieve:

- this week
- short term (within the next year)
- long term (within the next 5 years)
- lifetime
- any you might have completed already

Look at these final 10 and where they fit. What patterns do you see and notice?

From the final 10, shortlist them to 3 goals. It doesn't matter if they're short term or long term; these 3 goals are the ones I want you to focus on when reading this book.

Make a note of your 3 goals somewhere prominent you will see them. Maybe stick them on a noticeboard in your house. Pin them to the bathroom mirror so you can look at them every morning. Create a new screensaver for your phone with your top 3 goals in view.

Setting Your Smart Goals

Now you have your top 3 goals in mind; it's time to work on making them SMART.

Reading a book on self-discipline, then building action steps and habits to achieve your goals is pointless unless you have that right goal in mind.

Yet at the same time, keeping a goal in your mind is actually the very worst thing you can do.

Why?

A goal in mind is just a dream. You can dream and wish and want all day long but until you start creating some action steps to work on, that dream and your success will not move off the first step of the goal ladder.

Many years ago, I read a very famous book by Rhona Byrne, *The Secret*, which explains the power of The Law of Attraction and gratitude. You may have read it?

I consumed this book and read all her follow-up work. I started practising gratitude through journaling and even set up a successful Facebook group to get others to join in and feel grateful about many aspects of their lives.

I felt happier the whole time throughout this group gratitude challenge. So did the other people who joined me in this daily practice. It was powerful in changing how we thought and felt and enabled us to see positives in negative situations.

It was hard to feel negative and hard-done-by when we were being grateful for everything in our lives multiple times each day. However, I really didn't achieve all I'd been hoping to throughout the challenge and in the months afterwards

One recurrent theme in all of Rhonda Byrne's books is *Ask. Believe. Receive.*

She encourages you to "*ask* the Universe" for what you want, "*believe* it to be true, and act as if it has already happened" and then to "*receive* all that you desire" from the Universe.

I practised this for a couple of years. I made vision boards and meditated, visualising my goals in my mind. Some of my goals I did achieve. This simple practice had brought them into my consciousness, and I was now aware of the steps I had to take, and I took them quite naturally.

Other goals fell by the wayside. A simple matter of daydreaming about them wasn't going to help me focus my efforts and create a plan.

That's why I believe the '*Ask. Believe. Receive*' message is flawed. It is no good keeping your goals as pictures in your mind or on a vision board. Your goals need a strategy and a plan.

I am a big believer that the right and more realistic formula for achieving your goals in this realistic plan:

- Ask
- Believe
- Devise an action plan of small steps towards your goal

- Action these steps every single day
- Achieve

How Do You Devise an Action Plan for Your Goals?

Now we have your top 3 goals in mind, I encourage you to follow the SMART method when looking to devise a plan on how to achieve them. It will help you figure out exactly what you want and how to get there.

It follows this acronym:

- **S** - Specific
- **M** - Measurable
- **A** - Attainable
- **R** - Relevant
- **T** - Timely

I'll outline each one individually and a set of helpful questions you can ask yourself when goal setting.

SMART Goal Setting - Specific

Getting specific with your goal will help you decide what it is you actually want to achieve. The more specific you can be with your goal outline, the bigger chance you have of achieving it.

Throughout this book, I will pose various questions to you. These questions will appear with this word: >>>*Journal*<<<

It is a valuable exercise to get a notebook specifically for the work you will do alongside this book and make notes as you read. You can answer the questions and discover your own truth and path this way.

>>> *Journal* <<<

The following questions may help you get specific:

- What do I want to accomplish?
- Why do I want to achieve this?
- What do I need to stop doing?
- What do I need to start doing?
- What are the challenges?

SMART Goal Setting - Measurable

There's nothing worse than having a goal in mind, working on it and then changing the goalposts once you're on your way. Knowing your endpoint and at what point to pop open the Champagne is vital for feeling a sense of achievement.

You'll need to provide evidence to yourself for this section and a clear checklist to refine exactly what it is that you want. Defining this section will make your goal crystal clear and easy to reach.

>>> *Journal* <<<

Questions to think about:

- How will I measure my progress?
- How will I know when I have achieved this goal?

SMART Goal Setting - Attainable

It really IS possible to take a goal that seems impossible, plan smart and go for it at all costs until we achieve it. However, sometimes we also need to be a little realistic. Do we have the time? Do we have the talent? Do we have the money? Do we have the effort required for every step of the journey?

This section will help you to weigh up the time, effort and other costs your goal will take against the profits and other obligations and priorities you have in life.

The last thing you want to do is bankrupt yourself or end up divorced because of a seemingly possible goal.

There is absolutely nothing wrong with dreaming big and aiming for the moon when it comes to goals. Just add in a pinch of reality here when answering the following questions:

>>> *Journal* <<<

- How can this goal be accomplished?
- What are the logistical steps I can take?

SMART Goal Setting - Relevant

This one requires a lot of soul searching and thought. Is reaching this goal relevant to you or someone or something else?

Are you going for this for the right reasons? Will this make you and your family happier? Healthier?

Are you just going for this to show off, or for the validation and acceptance of others? Or is this something that truly makes your heart sing and gives you the tingles just thinking about it?

If you are lacking in certain skills or qualifications you can retrain. If you lack resources or finances, you can create a strategy to look for and secure them.

If you are lacking in time, with family commitments, then this is the section to explore that and what it will look like.

Do you really want to be famous, jetting around the world on your speaking tour with three kids at home and a partner who hasn't seen you for weeks?

>>> *Journal* <<<

Questions to ask yourself and the relevance of this goal:

- Is this a worthwhile goal?
- Is this the right time in my life?
- Do I have the necessary resources to accomplish this goal?
- Is this goal in line with my long-term objectives?

- How will this goal enhance my life?

SMART Goal Setting - Timely

Setting deadlines for yourself will turn your dreams into reality. Switching from dreaming to action requires a time-sensitive plan and a deadline for yourself, your team or anyone else involved in your goal. A plan will be the difference between success and failure.

Keep a realistic timeline and keep it flexible too - just in case any curveballs come your way. On the flip side, there would be nothing worse than wasting the launch of a product or service by going at it too soon, before it is ready. You don't want to be burning yourself and everyone else out as you race towards the finish line.

Keep morale high and check in regularly on those involved in your goal, or get yourself an accountability buddy who is working on their own project to bounce ideas off. We'll explore that in more detail in *Step 3 - Ways to Stay Accountable*.

>>> *Journal* <<<

Timely questions to ask yourself:

- How long will it take to accomplish this goal?
- When is the completion date of this goal?
- When am I going to work on this goal?

Making Goals SMART

Let's take three different hypothetical goals and make them SMART in the following examples.

1. I want to lose weight.
2. I want to be a millionaire.
3. I want to change career.

All three goals above are very vague and what we would refer to as 'passive' goals. Let's now make them SMART active goals with suggested specifics. These are example goals and not mine or linked to anyone in particular.

I Want to Lose Weight

S - Specific

What do I want to accomplish?
I want to lose at least 24lb of body fat.

Why do I want to achieve this?
Because none of my clothes fit me, and I am not feeling good about myself.

What do I need to stop doing?
Eating junk food, eating takeaways, drinking sugary drinks, consuming too much alcohol, making excuses about the gym.

What do I need to start doing?
Drink 2 litres of water a day, reduce my sugary drinks consumption, change my alcohol from beer to spirits and mixers and work on reducing consumption, going to the gym four times a week.

What are the challenges?
Cravings for sugary sweets, not preparing food in advance and eating out, no motivation for the gym, getting up too late.

M - Measurable

How will I measure my progress?
I will check in with myself each week. I will weigh myself and take measurements every Monday and take update pictures every four weeks.

How will I know when I have achieved this goal?
When I have lost 24lbs.

A - Attainable

How can this goal be accomplished?
By drinking water every day, reducing sugary drinks, reducing alcohol, going to the gym, getting up earlier, pushing myself harder when exercising.

What are the logistical steps I can take?

- I will prep my meals in advance to keep me on track
- I will buy myself a new water bottle and keep it with me
- I will install an app to track my water consumption
- I will aim for 10,000 steps each day on my Fitbit
- I will diarise my gym sessions every week in advance
- I will ask my friend to become my gym buddy and train with me
- I will keep track of my progress each week

R - Relevant

Is this a worthwhile goal?
Yes, I will feel healthier, look better and have more energy for other areas of my life. It will improve my self-confidence and prove to myself that I can achieve my goals.

Is this the right time?
Yes, there is no time like the present to work on my health and well-being.

Do I have the necessary resources to accomplish this goal?
Yes, I have a gym membership, but I could research home and bodyweight workouts I can do from anywhere so that I continue to train.

Is this goal in line with my long-term objectives?
Yes, long term, I want to be as healthy as possible to live a long and happy life.

T - Timely

How long will it take to accomplish this goal?
I will aim for 1lb per week, so 24 weeks.

When is the completion date of this goal?
24 weeks from now.

When am I going to work on this goal?

Every day with drinking water and nutrition and four times a week for the gym.

I Want to Be a Millionaire

S - Specific

What do I want to accomplish?
I want to earn a million dollars a year by creating a new app to help sales teams make more sales calls and make more money.

Why do I want to achieve this?
Because I believe I can and I know that this will help so many people to also achieve their business goals.

What do I need to stop doing?
Having self-doubt, believing that I "don't know enough", procrastinating, worrying about the finances.

What do I need to start doing?
Create a sustainable daily routine that factors in time to work on the app development. Recruit an investor to help with the finances. Recruit another developer to create the app.

What are the challenges?
Finances and not having enough investment. My own anxiety and overwhelm. My day-to-day business responsibilities, as this currently pays the bills and is a priority.

M - Measurable

How will I measure my progress?
I will get myself an accountability buddy and organise regular check-ins and conversations to keep me on track with my goal.

I will create a launch timeline, scheduling regular meetings and analysis of our progress.

How will I know when I have achieved this goal?
When my app is generating $84,000 dollars in paid revenue per month.

A - Attainable

How can this goal be accomplished?

- By creating a comprehensive strategy from idea development to implementation, marketing to maintenance.

- By recruiting investors to assist financially on the project.

- By identifying which team members can be responsible for each section.

- By creating team communication and benchmarks for each stage using software like Slack, Asana, Trello or Evernote.

What are the logistical steps I can take?

- I will create a full outline of the app, the content and how it works.

- I will create a presentation about the inner workings of the app to present to investors.

- I will recruit an accountability buddy to keep me on track with my goals and bounce ideas off.

- I will recruit another developer to share the workload and create the app software.

- I will plan and write a book about sales alongside the app to help promote the app.

- I will recruit copywriters to create valuable content on sales tips for social media and blogs to help drive traffic towards downloading the app once developed.

R - Relevant

Is this a worthwhile goal?
Yes, this is something I have wanted to achieve for a long time and will enable me to help many people at once while creating a passive income.

Is this the right time?
Yes, there are many apps on the market. I have downloaded most of them, and they fall short in terms of keeping me on track. I believe I have the right model to help people not only establish effective sales accountability but maintain it.

Do I have the necessary resources to accomplish this goal?
I have around 75% of the resources to achieve this goal at present with my own knowledge, research and content. I am lacking in funding and know with time constraints that I should consider hiring another developer to move the project along quicker.

Is this goal in line with my long-term objectives?
Yes, my long-term objective is to earn $1m a year, and this goal will help me achieve that.

T - Timely

How long will it take to accomplish this goal?
I will aim to set up the app in one year and achieve my revenue income goal within the next five years.

When is the completion date of this goal?
One year from now for the app, and five years from now for the financial goal.

When am I going to work on this goal?
I am going to use the first 60 minutes of my day to work on this goal Monday to Friday and plan a whole day once a month on the weekend to work on this goal.

This will give me a minimum of 28 hours per month to work on this goal.

I Want to Change My Career

S - Specific

What do I want to accomplish?
I want to be a highly successful qualified personal trainer.

Why do I want to achieve this?
Because I am unhappy and unfulfilled in my current role and I have wanted a career change for a long time.

What do I need to stop doing?
Wasting time on social media, worrying about paying the bills, delaying starting my training.

What do I need to start doing?
Commit to a training course, decide on a timescale for study, diary in practice and theory study.

What are the challenges?
Studying while working full time.

M - Measurable

How will I measure my progress?
I will check in with myself each week to assess how my study has gone. I will ask a close friend to be someone I can answer to and who I will tell when I have completed study and assignments.

How will I know when I have achieved this goal?
When I achieve my qualification, leave my job to become a personal trainer AND have a diary full of paying clients.

A - Attainable

How can this goal be accomplished?
By committing time to study and practice.

What are the logistical steps I can take?

- I will get up 1 hour earlier every day to study over breakfast and coffee.
- I will dedicate 3 hours each Saturday and Sunday morning to my study or practical learning in the gym.
- I will regularly assess myself and my progress, making sure I am not procrastinating and falling behind.
- I will contact personal trainers I know and ask to shadow them for a day or two.
- I will book annual leave and book in a time to shadow other personal trainers.
- I will start to make contact with gyms and local personal trainer companies to secure a role at the end of my training.
- I will look into marketing for fitness professionals to help me market myself

once I am qualified.

R - Relevant

Is this a worthwhile goal?
Yes, I want a career change, and I have always wanted to do this.

Is this the right time?
Yes, I am not getting any younger, and I am very unhappy in my current job.

Do I have the necessary resources to accomplish this goal?
Yes, I have signed up to the course, I have my course materials and study, and there is a wealth of information out there for me to read up on in addition to my course study.

Is this goal in line with my long-term objectives?
Yes, I am very excited about a career that will not only fulfil me but keep me healthy and happy too.

T - Timely

How long will it take to accomplish this goal?
My course is three months long, so I am to hand in my notice at work in 8 weeks and have secured a position within a gym setting by the time my course finishes.

When is the completion date of this goal?
Three months from now.

When am I going to work on this goal?
Every morning over breakfast, bedtime reading on evenings where I have more free time and 3 hours every Saturday and Sunday for reading and practical study.

I will also book annual leave before I leave my job to shadow other fitness professionals and seek their knowledge and guidance.

Focus on the Positive

One thing that is vital when setting SMART goals is to formulate a positive plan of action.

It's all about what you focus ON, and that will increase. When you focus on NOT doing something that is often the 'thing' you end up concentrating on.

So instead of telling yourself that you will 'stop feeling overwhelmed' for example, you can flip that and instead say 'create a daily focused action plan'.

Another example, instead of telling yourself 'tomorrow I will stop eating chocolate', you can flip it to a positive and productive behaviour instead and say 'tomorrow I will drink more water and take more fruit for my snack'.

Assess Along the Way

Make sure you take time to assess your goals along the way. At the start of any SMART goal process, you might want to diarise specific time slots over the course of the goal duration to check in with yourself.

For example, if you have given yourself a 12-week timeframe for your goal, pop a reminder in your diary every week or two weeks to assess how you are doing with your goal and if you are working on the right things at that time to move you forward.

Do those diary reminders now. In advance. They make a difference.

We will talk about assessing your progress and checking in on yourself throughout your goal journey in more depth in *Step 8 - The Weekly Check-in Process*.

Know When to Stop and Reward

Planning in rewards and moments to celebrate your goal achievements are very important. In Shawn Acor's brilliant book, *The Happiness Advantage*, and subsequent TED talk on this subject, Shawn discovers that human beings make themselves miserable when they change their pre-set goal posts that define success.

As a Harvard professor in Positive Psychology, Shawn has helped people all over the world to improve their productivity and performance by over 30%.

How? He focused on happiness. His work took him to over 42 countries and working within schools and companies all over the world. Each place he went, he asked his crowd what was the formula for happiness that had been taught to them from childhood? The answer was usually the same:

Work hard = be successful = be happy.

But this formula is flawed and broken. For every time we achieve success, we then move the goalposts and expect happiness to be on the other side of that. So effectively we are always chasing happiness and never feel fulfilled.

Let's use someone working in a sales role as an example of this.

If Jeff hits his sales target for the last quarter, his target for the next quarter gets increased. That's just the way of the sales world. Yet this is extremely frustrating for Jeff. One way this is combatted is by commission or a sales bonus; Jeff is financially rewarded for achieving his target however that target changes constantly and the job gets harder and harder with every new goal post that is changed and repositioned.

Along the way of your goal journey, it is important to stop and assess every micro success. This will keep you motivated and fuel you onwards to continue with the daily steps needed to achieve your goal.

Once you have set the end goal and the time limit - STICK TO IT! If you said you wanted to lose 10lb, then celebrate when you lose 10lb! Don't decide that it isn't enough and that you now actually want to lose 10lb more.

You might want to treat yourself when you reach these goals, a little like Jeff's bonus. You might treat yourself to a new outfit if you lose a dress size, or a mini-break if you achieve sales of $3000 a month, for example. Just know what it is you're achieving and make sure you have a plan to celebrate it when you get there.

We go into more depth on this in Chapter 9.

Getting Clear on What You Want

I worked on the first version of this book during downtime while watching a friend of mine compete in a bodybuilding show.

It's the first time he had done something like this. At 33 years of age, he had spent the last eight years working as a fitness coach and before that, had hopes of competing as a professional boxer. Sadly, the boxing career wasn't to be, and a hand injury and subsequent operation meant he had to hang up his gloves for good. Yet that ingrained desire and drive to compete, to win, has never really left him.

He decided to try out for a bodybuilding show to have some element of healthy competition in his life again, now that his professional boxing career is no more. He said that he would use the training months to compete with himself, and then on the day of the show it would feel like a boxing match; him against his opponents (the other competitors on stage).

He competed with himself because of a deep-rooted desire to prove to himself that he had what it takes. Because he was so clear on what he wanted, the process was relatively easy - even when restricting his calorie intake as drastically as he did. His clarity on his goal, coupled with his self-discipline and daily habits meant he emerged victorious and not only won his category, but the overall show too.

It was wonderful inspiration for me, and timely when writing this book. There were over 150 men and women on that bodybuilding stage that weekend who all possessed the most incredible levels of self-discipline and self-control – particularly around food and training.

Each bodybuilding competitor on that stage was in the most incredible condition and had worked hard for months, sometimes years, to get to their goal. Their consistent daily habits in terms of food and training paid off on the day.

I overheard one woman at the show who was struggling mentally with the final show day stress. All she could talk about was her need for doughnuts at the end of the show. She also said "I'll show them. Who's had the last laugh now?!" She then started a conversation with her friends, and it turned out that this woman was bullied as a child for being overweight. This was the drive that had got her in the competition-ready muscular shape she was in. She was obsessed with getting pictures for social media and was all smiles for the camera, yet when the lens was away from her face, she looked entirely miserable!

So with the two scenarios above, which one is clear on their 'why' and which one is possibly attempting this for the wrong reasons?

I'm not saying that the woman couldn't go out there and give it her all, achieving an amazing goal, but is it really the right reason? If you're looking to achieve a goal to get a sense of validation, or please someone else, or to fight back against demons from your past, is that goal true to you? And true to you as a person here and now in this present moment?

Being Honest About Why You Want It

Knowing the reason behind your motivation to do something, or achieve a goal is a challenge, but can give you a great indication whether you will follow through with your goal or not.

After all, if you're not working towards a goal for the right reasons, you're more likely to forget about it, drop it, or worse - hate the process!

So it's time to get ridiculously honest with yourself.

>>> Journal <<<

Take a minute to ask yourself the following questions:

- What is my driving force behind this goal?
- How will this goal positively impact my life?
- How will this goal negatively impact my life?
- What will I need to give up in my life to achieve this goal?
- Am I prepared to do that?
- What will I need to add to my life to achieve this goal?
- What do those I love think of this goal?
- Is this goal for me and me only, or am I really doing this to please/impress someone else?
- How will my life change once I have reached this goal?

Have a good look back at your answers and see what you said to yourself. If you feel like this goal truly is for you, and you know this will positively impact your life, then it is time to embark on those self-discipline hacks and habits to get you there.

Part 2

The 10 Steps to Stop Procrastinating And Achieve Your Goals

Step 1

Establishing Your Solid Morning Routine

"You will never change your life until you change something you do daily. The secret of your success is found in your daily routine."
– Unknown (stolen from Instagram!)

"Gemma you can't just tell people to get up early. Nobody wants to get up early. We need to tell people why it is so powerful and works, and let them decide whether it is worth getting up early for."

Said Ben. My book buddy (you'll hear more about how our little accountability buddy arrangement works in *Step 5 – Ways to Stay Accountable*).

Ben was right. The first draft of this book basically told you to get up early and follow a morning routine. Which I will still tell you about in a minute. First I want to let you in on a secret.

The secret is, it's *no secret* that any book, podcast, article or interview with a successful CEO, entrepreneur, innovator that you listen to or read, they say the same thing when asked that same question about the secret of their success. It wasn't overnight, it wasn't handed to them on a plate, they worked for it, and they worked hard. The likes of Robin Sharma, Tony Robbins, Oprah Winfrey, all belong to the same club.

A club? There's a secret club, you say? How do I get in? You *can. Anyone can*. It's the early morning club. But one with a conscious set of self-discipline actions so powerful, they can change your life.

On New Year's Day 2016, I read an article from the New York Times about a journalist who had read two books that changed her life.

The first was Marie Kondo, *The Life-Changing Magic of Tidying Up* and the second Hal Elrod, *The Miracle Morning*.

The Life-Changing Magic of Tidying Up is a manual on how to get rid of clutter in your life, stop buying stuff you don't need and find joy in everything you own.

The Miracle Morning is a manual on how to get up early and complete six different tasks in six specific categories to help you level up your life.

In the article, this woman stood looking lithe and shiny in skin and hair, draped smugly across the furniture of her clean, organised, minimalist and calming home. She'd picked up both books the year before and had been following both manuals for a whole year. The article was her sharing the results of living life by the two manuals. She told tales of her financial triumphs, how she'd saved thousands by not buying stuff to clutter her home. She wrote in beautiful heartfelt prose about the calmness of her mornings thanks to Hal Elrod's methods and how she felt like a new person, in a permanent zen-like mode of stress-free wonderfulness. I was hooked on her every word. How the hell had she done this?

And then the biggest shock of all. Right there, at the end of the article, there she was, pictured with her two boys. Two twin toddler boys. She oozed that super mum smug look from every freshly moisturised pore.

I put the article down. Looked at my absolute tip of a house, my muffin top, my overdraft and I sighed a heavy heartfelt sigh. I wanted her life. I wanted it all.

I downloaded both books. As it was New Year, I had a week off work, and instead of bingeing on box sets and chocolate selection boxes, I consumed every word. I watched YouTube tutorials, and I read blog after blog on the art of tidying and the magic of waking up early.

By the time I went back to work a week later my house was unrecognisable and clutter-free. I'd lost half a stone. I'd sold a load of stuff on eBay and was back in the black.

The most significant difference was how I felt and how I behaved in the morning. I was getting up to do the routine around 90 minutes earlier than I had been.

Hal Elrod's *Miracle Morning* concept is you follow six specific actions in the morning using the easy-to-remember acronym: SAVERS. They include things like meditation, affirmations, visualising yourself a success, exercise, reading and journaling.

It's a brilliant little book that gets you to create a solid morning routine with these specific actions you can follow.

Reading *The Miracle Morning* and applying the knowledge gleaned from the book allowed me to take responsibility for my actions. I successfully turned my mornings into a productive powerhouse of activity that empowered me to change my whole life.

You see, up until that point I'd convinced myself that I was not a morning person and there's no way I could get up early every day. In my early twenties, I'd had a job as a radio presenter on the breakfast shift that required me to get up at 5 am. I struggled for years and years to get up. I would tell everyone who listened how exhausted I was all the time, and even likened my early mornings to feeling like I had "constant jetlag".

I can now tell you that was fabricated and in my own head.

I allowed myself to continually complain about tiredness and tell myself that I COULDN'T get up on time every day. It got so bad that I referred myself to a sleep disorder centre, convinced there was something medically wrong with me.

Years later, after countless frustrating mornings of stress, lateness and never feeling prepared for my day, I picked up *The Miracle Morning* and within 24 hours of reading the book, I couldn't believe I was getting up 90 mins earlier than I usually would be, with ease.

Why? I took responsibility for my own thoughts, and I told myself I *could*.

I recommend *The Miracle Morning* to so many people, and it's usually met with an "I honestly can't get up in the morning" response. I promise you can learn to love mornings.

The Purpose of the Morning Routine

Your morning routine is created to make your life easier and help you start your day on the right foot.

If you create time for yourself in the morning and the things that will help energise you, you will start your day with a spring in your step and feel in control.

Before I focused on my morning routine, ahead of my working day, my mornings were insane. My husband leaves for work at 7 am, and I would always sleep in. I'd set multiple alarms in different places around the house, and I'd sleep through them all. Eventually, I'd wake from my slumber and then run around like a woman possessed to get me and my son ready, and then off to school on time. It was horrible, stressful and every morning saw me shouting and cursing until we were out of the door - especially at my son who was only just five years old at this point.

I wasn't proud of my behaviour, and I knew it was not his fault at all. I was screaming at him to put socks on or hurry up eating his breakfast, but he's just a kid with no concept of time, and he's my responsibility. I'd shout and stress from the moment I opened my eyes. I'd get him into school, late of course, and then I'd have to sprint, not run but sprint (often in heels!) to get to my train on time. I would regularly go to work in tears.

Something had to change.

I found the morning routine and my life did change. I started my day with silent calm. I carved out valuable solitary time for myself. I began to move my body and feel like I had more energy. I loved writing about my feelings and emptying my head into my journal. It was a complete contrast from what life had been like for years. My mornings finally became my favourite part of my day and a true gift. Yours can too if your morning sounds even a smidge as stressful as mine did.

Starting Your Morning Routine

If you aren't an all or nothing person like me, I'd recommend starting small when starting your morning routine.

You're more likely to stick to something if you start small and work your way up. Go all-in straight away, and you'll just give up and go back to old and comfortable habits.

Think about your mornings and the things you enjoy doing, or the things you know you could incorporate into your life that will benefit you. Exercise, meditation, keeping a gratitude journal, eating a healthy breakfast are all examples of things you might want to start fitting into your life.

Now let's start with 5 minutes only.

If you've woken up later than ever, the proverbial has hit the fan, what one thing can you do in minutes or seconds that will help your day go better?

Mine is to make a proper coffee and while it's pouring (takes 1 min 31 seconds - I timed it!) I can take some really deep breaths, and I can stretch. This makes a difference in how I feel if I am running a little late. It helps me stave off the stress, take a minute to focus and make a conscious decision of how my morning will play out. I love a cup of coffee to start my day and calming myself with some deep breathing, stretching my arms and core is better than doing nothing at all and staying in a stressed state, and it takes mere minutes.

What could you do in five minutes that would help you feel centred, feel in control and feel like you've reclaimed the morning? Something that will put you on the right foot for the day, even if it only takes less than five minutes?

I asked readers for help with this one, and here are some of their suggestions for five-minute actions in the morning:

- The conscious choice to know that I don't have the time to check any of my notifications on my phone, put it by the door and focus on getting ready
- Putting on my makeup and a pair of heels
- A quick yoga sequence
- Ten jumping jacks
- A five-minute meditation
- Saying aloud three things I am grateful for
- Sitting still for five minutes and visualising a smooth and stress-free morning with no traffic!
- Stroking my dog

- Having a swift cold shower to invigorate me and wake me up properly so I'll move quickly and get out on time
- Putting on my favourite song and dancing like crazy
- Reading an inspirational quote
- Adult colouring book time
- Saying my prayers and asking God to help me have a great day

What about you? Can you write down a list of things you could easily do in five minutes or less each morning to put you in a calm and positive state-of-mind?

Now repeat this and create some actions and activities for your morning if you had:

- 15 minutes available
- 30 minutes available
- 45 minutes available
- 60 minutes available
- 60+ minutes available

You can even use the above method to train yourself to get up earlier gradually. Start with setting your alarm 5 minutes earlier in the first week, 15 minutes in the second, 30 minutes in the third and so on.

Please do not feel that you must wake up over 60 minutes earlier than you usually do. You do not need to get up at 5 am to be a success. Having a healthy balance of great quality sleep and a morning routine will make a world of difference to how you feel each day. Be realistic with what will work for you, your routine, your lifestyle, your family dynamic and your personal energy levels. Don't sacrifice sleep for 'the hustle'. You'd be better focusing your efforts on sleeping earlier than getting up earlier if you do want to aim for that 5 am get up time.

Ideas for Your Morning Routine

A morning routine needs to be enjoyable for you; otherwise, like anything, you won't stick to it. Consistency is the key here, so carving out your own golden time in the morning doing stuff you love is worth it.

Here's what I'd recommend personally to incorporate into a morning routine:

Meditation

Meditation or quiet reflection is a great way to get your brain to rest and listen to your thoughts each morning. You can ask yourself deep questions and think of answers in meditation or mindfulness practise, or choose to sit in silence and reflect.

Download a meditation app that can take you through guided systematic meditations depending on your need. For example, if you suffer from anxiety, there is an anxiety meditation package in the Headspace app which you can follow.

One app I love is Insight Timer. At the time of publishing the first edition of this book, the app was free, but that isn't the case anymore. Much like many apps on the market now, Insight Timer operates a subscription fee that is paid monthly or annually. Or you can choose to pay for different meditation courses. I pay for the annual membership and feel that it is worth it. I use the app for focused music for working and even use the meditation for children courses with my son. You can choose all sorts of meditation audio packages and courses on a range of subjects, or use the timed feature for sitting in silence and meditating with the option of choosing humming, water or other sound effects in the background.

The trick with mindfulness or meditation is to allow thoughts to come in, honour them, and then let them go. Focus on your breathing and your body and sit in the moment.

If you practise meditation regularly, you will see a considerable shift in your motivation and decision-making becomes easier. You will start to notice your emotions and responses more, you will ask yourself powerful questions (for we all have the answers within us) and you will feel more centred, calm and less stressed.

It is also a great time just to be still and be. It's a moment of calm, devoid of the hustle and bustle of everyday life. If you commute to your job, have kids or a generally manic schedule you will start to relish these silent moments in the morning. Many people call this time 'golden hour' and they're not wrong.

A Moment of Morning Mindfulness

If you have tried meditating and just can't get to grips with it, try this easy to remember morning mindfulness moment. I always recommend sitting still in the morning, ideally with a lovely warm cup of tea or coffee. Just sit with the cup in your hands and focus on the following sensations:

Touch
Feel the cup's warmth in your hands or the feel of the cup's texture. Notice how your body and skin feels against the clothing you are wearing, the texture of the chair in which you are sitting, the feeling of your feet on the ground.

Sight
Focus on the hot drink in front of you and what you can see in your peripheral vision. What do you notice?

Sound
What can you hear as you notice the feel of the cup in your hand and the vision of the steam rising up? What sounds are around you right now in this moment?

Smell
Bring the cup closer to your nose and take a deep breath. What does your drink smell like? Bring the cup down and take another long, deep breath. What scents are you experiencing at this moment?

Taste
Finally, as long as it's not too hot, take a sip of your drink. What are your taste buds reporting? What does it actually taste like to you at this moment?

This process only takes a few minutes, but it allows you to focus on one thing and be completely present and mindful in the moment. There's no pressure to meditate and stop those thoughts coming in and out of your mind. You just focus on your warm drink and your senses. It is a calming exercise and will help you enter your day in a soothed state of mind.

Positive Affirmations

An affirmation is a declaration or statement that you make to affirm something.

Personal affirmations you repeat to yourself are extremely valuable and help you connect to what you want. Positive affirmations are short statements that are used to reprogram your thought patterns and change how you feel about things. They allow you to focus on goals, get rid of negative thoughts, change beliefs and program the subconscious mind.

Deciding on affirmations and the way you repeat them to yourself causes debate. Many will tell you to make these statements as if they have already happened or believe them to be happening and true (even if they aren't). In this case, you would start an affirmation with "I am".

For example:

- I am powerful
- I am beautiful
- I am healthy
- I am a champion
- I am smoke-free
- I am strong and lean

Other professionals believe that stating affirmations with "I am" may not be believable for the person speaking the words and instead advise to start affirmations with "I intend to" or "I will".

Whether you use "I am..." or "I intend to...", include these elements when choosing the words for your affirmation:

Speaking in the Present Tense

If you are able to feel like this is happening in the here and now, that you will have or can be something, then it is more likely to happen. Stating your affirmation in the future may just keep it there - in the future and out of reach.

Keep It Positive

Affirmations should state what you want, not what you don't want. Using positive sentences instead of negative will have powerful repercussions. If you don't want a situation, like you may want to stop smoking, instead of saying "I intend to stop smoking" say: "I am smoke-free" or "I am a non-smoker".

Does It Feel Good?

Notice your emotions when you say your affirmations. Do they feel good? Do they bring up good feelings? Or do they make you feel worried and anxious? They should make you feel good, and you should believe in them strongly.

Other examples of affirmations could be:

The "I am" way

- I am working less and earning more
- I am the world champion
- I am healthy and strong with muscle definition
- I am organised and productive
- I am a money magnet, and money flows into my life effortlessly
- I am healthy and strong and live life to the fullest
- I am forgiving and loving
- I love who I am and am happy in my skin

The "I intend to" way

- I intend to reduce my hours and spend more time with the children
- I intend to take responsibility for all my actions
- I intend to live with courage
- I intend to be self-assured and self-confident
- I intend to enjoy my life with enthusiasm
- I intend to have a positive attitude towards difficult circumstances
- I intend to let the people in my life know that they are important to me
- I intend to forgive myself lovingly for the mistakes I make
- I intend to live a fulfilling life and enrich other people's lives

Carrie Green, who runs the highly successful Female Entrepreneur Association, has her daily affirmation that starts a little different, but it makes you think! "I can, and I will. Watch me." Carrie's affirmation is a good example of a mantra for when you're striving for something that others might deem impossible.

Reciting Affirmations

Affirmations can be recited back to yourself or written down.

The most powerful way to recite affirmations is to speak them aloud to yourself while looking in a mirror. The mirror technique requires you to look yourself in the eye and say the affirmations aloud, speaking to your subconscious and conscious self. It is genuinely life-changing when this is performed. You cannot lie to yourself in the mirror, and your affirmations will be burned into your subconscious, making you more likely to live them out.

You could journal your affirmations, or you could put them on cards or prominent places around your home so that you will see them regularly.

You can even purchase affirmation cards. Louise L Hay's *Power Thought Cards* are a great choice for this and very handy to have. If you're struggling for affirmation inspiration, you can draw a card from the deck and see if it fits with you and your own goals. I also recommend Brendon Burchard's *The Motivation Manifesto Cards* for affirmations that feel more serious and less spiritual.

Visualising Your Goal Achievements

Dream it, and you can become it!

Much like affirmations, visualisation takes it one step further and gets you to imagine your goal or statements as if they have already happened.

Did you know? Your brain does not know the difference between what is real and what is imagined. It is the reason why a vivid dream can feel so real, and sometimes why you question past events and wonder if you have imagined them, or if they were reality.

With that in mind, visualising success is a very important and widely used tool to teach the brain what you want in life and form those neural pathways to make it happen.

Many professional athletes use positive psychology and visualisation to imagine the feeling of winning that Olympic gold, or scoring that winning goal. There is much money spent on the mental conditioning of professional athletes, and visualisations play a considerable role.

What do you want? By now, you should know what your goal is. Don't forget about the Goal Setting Masterclass I have gifted you as part of this book. If you are yet to watch it and download the workbook, you can do so here: **www.gemmaray.com/bonus**.

>>>*Journal*<<<

With your goal(s) in mind, take a moment, maybe at the end of your meditation or mindfulness practise to really visualise your situation as if it is already happening right now.

- What can you see?
- What can you hear?
- What can you smell?
- What can you taste?
- What do you look like?
- How do you feel?
- Where are you?

Remember all those tiny details and focus on that end goal. If you're looking to lose weight, how are you looking and feeling? What are you wearing? What are others saying about your success?

If you're looking for financial success, how much is on your bank statement? What are you able to buy now that you're financially successful? How much money do you have in your hands?

If you're aiming for that promotion at work, what does it feel like knowing you've achieved it? What is your new office like? What does your new suit or clothing feel and look like? How are you feeling and acting in your new role?

You can even use visualisations in your affirmation work. If you are making positive statements that you can imagine happening in the present, say it aloud to yourself, look in the mirror and then take a moment to visualise that it is already happening for you.

Your brain is constantly scanning the environment every single second, and while the primary function is to keep you alive and safe, it also looks for opportunities.

If you're telling yourself every day that you want a promotion, your brain will look for those opportunities in your working life that can help you step up and make that visualisation a reality. An overheard conversation, an email, a way to prove yourself; your brain will bring these into your consciousness to match up with all you have been visualising.

Get Your Blood Pumping!

Moving your body first thing in the morning fires up your brain, your blood flow and your muscles. After a night in bed, getting up and getting moving is a great way to start your day.

Getting it out of the way at the start of the day works well for some people. You just do it and don't have to think about it! When researching this book, I came across people who swore by going to bed in their gym clothes, they just got up and got out - before their brain had a chance to argue back! That's one way of doing it.

Whatever you do, just get moving. Some people grab their trainers and head straight out for a run. Some go off for a swim, and others do yoga. Some complete exercises at home or light stretches. You know your own abilities and limits, and the point is to just move and fire up your system.

Whatever you choose to do, the harder you can push yourself, the better. Exercise has been scientifically proven to improve lifestyle, mental health and reduce body fat among other amazing benefits.

If you need some convincing of the power of exercise, check out Dr Wendy Suzuki's 2017 TED Talk: *The Brain Changing Benefits of Exercise* about the immediate positive benefit of exercise on the brain for your mood and focus. She also details the protective benefits of exercise on the brain for conditions such as depression, dementia and other neurological conditions.

Learn/Read/Listen

How much new information do you learn every day? The infinite amount of research and knowledge at our disposal online and in print means you can self-study absolutely any topic you like.

Once you start on a self-development path, your eyes will be opened up to the multitude of life-changing and inspirational books, podcasts and online resources that will help motivate you. Your knowledge increases to help you excel in your chosen field and improve many different areas of your life.

In the book *Slight Edge* by Jeff Olsen, he points out that if the average book is 300 pages long, if you were to read ten pages of a book each day, you would read a book a month and that's 12 books a year.

Imagine how much extra knowledge and learning you could absorb by reading an additional 12 books in a year! Yet many of us see a book and think "Nah, haven't got time".

Of course, reading is not limited to books. The internet is a wealth of valuable information. You may choose to read articles, blogs or educational and motivational stories online. It all counts.

Remember, just ten pages or 10 minutes a day and all those extra books you could read. How much additional knowledge could you stockpile in a year? How would that impact your personal growth and self-development?

Keeping a Journal

I think there's something so powerful about writing things down in your handwriting.

In my Level Up community on Facebook, we chat about journaling a lot. Some people choose to journal and write a daily diary. Others choose to write out their affirmations and others choose to use the time to write out their intentions for the day: a to-do list of sorts.

Whichever way you choose to journal, it needn't take long. Putting pen to paper and seeing your own goals written down in your handwriting all helps cement that belief that you will, and *can* achieve your goal.

How Long Should My Morning Routine Take?

The duration of your morning routine is personal to you and also might change as you increase the strength of your self-discipline actions.

You still need to sleep and rest, and you may choose to start small, as suggested earlier in the chapter. Start with five minutes and start with the smallest action step. Build it up and see how you get on.

I am up 90 minutes to 2 hours before the rest of my family, and I choose to go to bed a little earlier to fit it all in. I've tried all sorts of adaptations of the morning routine. I did a 4 am morning for a long time before realising it wasn't working for me, and I was exhausted. My morning routine is not rigid and set-in-stone these days. My sleep is really important to me so I aim for a disciplined 10:00 pm bedtime and a 5:15 am get-up if it is a gym day and a 6 am get-up if not. My life has changed for the better since I adopted this approach, and my days are so productive and focused.

But that's me. That's not you. You will know your own body and sleeping patterns the best. If you don't, start to take notice. There are no rules with morning routines at all. You have to pick what works for you, but do give it a few weeks to test it and get used to whatever time you choose to wake up and start your morning routine.

Help! I Can't Get Up!

Oh, I hear you! Even now, I still really struggle to get up on that first alarm and snoozing the alarm is the most common objection and challenge for people I speak to who want to establish a better morning routine. I have a few alarms dotted around the house, including a Lumie clock which emulates sunset and sunrise to trick my brain into getting up. It's particularly helpful during the dark winter months. I also stopped charging my phone by my bed a few years ago as I realised it was too close to me and that was why I snoozed it every day.

Knowing this had been an issue for a long time for me, plus wanting to focus on getting more sleep and not staying up late scrolling, I made a pact with myself to always keep my phone downstairs at night time. In order to help me have more of a chance of succeeding in getting up without snoozing, I invested in a Geemarc alarm clock which is specifically designed for hearing imparied or heavy sleepers. It features a 95db alarm, flashing light and vibrating pad that goes under your pillow. I use the sound and light features and keep the alarm clock in the kitchen. It is placed there on purpose as I have to quickly get out of bed and come to the kitchen to turn it off before my son and husband wake up! As I have left the warmth and comfort of my bed to head downstairs to turn it off, it gives my brain the time

I need to wake up and start my morning routine.

As I am someone who has found getting up a real challenge, I've got lots of tips and hacks that I have tried and tested over the years that may help you get up in the morning:

Getting Up on Time – the Night Before Routine

For me, my morning routine starts the night before. I find if I do a download of the day in my head or journal and take a moment to plan out the following day, it helps me go to bed and sleep quicker with less on my mind.

Journaling the day's events is helpful as it feels like I'm emptying my head on paper. I also use the time to work out what I have coming up in the diary the next day and what my priorities are. Doing this helps me sometimes set that alarm a little earlier, or a little later and be more realistic about the time I have available the next day to achieve everything I've written down.

I find that there are often small 2/3 minute jobs that appear on this 'night before' list that I can tackle there and then. Sending that email, ordering that birthday present online, transferring a bit of money into the savings, putting away laundry or making our lunches are all examples of quick things that don't take long. Still, if they're off the list, the list feels lighter. Getting some of the small stuff off the list often feels like a significant achievement, and I'm winning before the night is over and the next morning has begun.

The Dress Rehearsal

If I've had a run of particularly rubbish mornings and I've not been able to get up, I actively visualise my morning by doing a night before 'dress rehearsal'. Hear me out on this one and humour me for a moment because I am well aware that what I am about to tell you sounds ludicrous. Try it though - it works!

I like to call this the dress rehearsal. At night, just before bedtime, I lie down in my bed and close my eyes, pretending to be asleep. I visualise my alarm clock going off. I close my eyes and visualise the alarm time displaying my get-up time. I picture myself seeing this time clearly on the alarm display as I sit up and swing my legs out of bed. I visualise tapping the alarm STOP button as I rise out of bed and start to walk to my door.

I pick up my dressing gown, put it on and walk to the bathroom. I splash my face with cold water, look in the mirror and say to myself in my head "Morning! Well done for getting up!" I then walk out of my bedroom, walk downstairs, let out my dogs (because it's bedtime and they need to pee anyway!), take three deep breaths as I open the front door to let them out into the fresh air and stretch.

Sometimes I repeat this dress rehearsal process 2 or 3 times. I then find that in the morning, when the alarm goes off, I know EXACTLY what to do (even though I have done this routine many times before). The dress rehearsal reminds me of the process and just how easy it is. It is the choice to hit snooze or stop, and the action steps I take straight after to keep me awake.

I know that sounds completely and utterly crazy but if you're someone who really struggles to get up each morning, give it a try and let me know if it works!

The Night Time Meditation

With the dress rehearsal above, if I have a spare 5 minutes, I'll try a quick meditation which incorporates the mantra "I love my mornings and waking up early." I try and do this before bed to put my mind in the right state to wake early. I also sometimes listen to subliminal recordings overnight (you can find these on YouTube) which help me wake up early.

Alarm Clocks from Hell

The number one way I get up early is using alarm clocks. I always have a minimum of two, sometimes more, but when I complete the dress rehearsal and meditation above, I usually get up on the first one and the rest act as insurance.

I write notes to myself on the phone and iPad that display as the alarm sounds. Sometimes I use inspirational quotes, sometimes I write some pretty lovely things to myself and other times I'm not so nice; "Get up you lazy cow!" is one that is quite effective!

I have also downloaded many apps in my time to help me get up. Some of them required me to take a picture in a specific spot or complete maths puzzles to wake up. All were really good, but I found I got clever quite quickly and even in my dozy state I work out ways to override their deafening instructions.

Recently I've discovered the most hilarious and irritating alarm app called Carrot. It spits insults out at me along with using mind bending puzzles and instructions to silence its deafening fog-horn like shrill. Just make sure your phone is plugged in and you leave the app running, otherwise it does tend to fail.

Making Mornings Work for You – Recap

Remember – start small! Start with just five minutes and set some realistic expectations of what you could do in that time. If you want to get up earlier in the morning try to set your alarm for 5 minutes earlier for a week. Then the week after set it for 10 minutes, and another 15 minutes the week after that. It will feel like less of a shock to the system!

Step 2

Make Your Health a Habit

"Your body isn't a temple. It is a home you will live in forever. Take care of it."
- Unknown

"Your health is your wealth" is a great thought-provoking statement that is undoubtedly true. You can have the flashiest car, the biggest house, the biggest bank account but none of it is as precious and important as the body you live in. It really is the only place you have to reside in this life.

The only certainty in life is death. Yet, figuratively speaking, the time when that happens can be extended due to a few factors.

I always start with this one early on, because no matter what your SMART goal may be, creating some healthy habits is universally recognised as a pillar of success. If you're overweight, unhealthy, stressed or not sleeping, you're not going to perform at your optimum levels.

Looking after your health is one of the fundamental habits that every goal-striving person should put first.

It is no good aiming for your first million-pound business if you're not feeling brilliant, not sleeping, stressed to death and living a miserable existence in your own body.

Prioritising your health means you will perform at your best.

How many people do you know who are too busy to drink water during the day, or take a lunch break? Heck, you might even be one of those people yourself!

Nobody is ever too busy for their health. It is a bullshit statement, and it just re-affirms the fact that you are putting yourself last and not prioritising your health.

Women are terrible at putting themselves first. Especially those women who have children. They prioritise everyone else's needs above their own and end up exhausted and fed up.

The first healthy habit to adopt is to PUT YOURSELF AND YOUR HEALTH FIRST.

Surviving off coffee and takeaways as you slave away on your goal will most certainly have a detrimental effect on your cognition and motivation.

If you want to remain super productive and with a laser-like focus at all times then the key to this is your health.

In this book, I encourage you to seriously consider the following to benefit your health and perform at your optimum best.

1. Drink at least 2 litres of water a day
2. Make conscious food choices and opt for whole single ingredient foods
3. Move your body
4. Look after your mental health
5. Develop a strict sleep hygiene routine

So let's look at each in more depth.

1. Drink 2 Litres of Water a Day

When looking at self-discipline with health I start on the good old H20. Water is the elixir of life and one really simple key habit of well-being that produces such powerful results when consumed in the right quantities.

Our bodies are made up of over 60 per cent water. Blood is 92 per cent water, the brain and muscles around 75 per cent water and bones around 22 per cent water.

Water regulates your body temperature, lubricates joints, protects the spine and other tissues, and acts as the primary mechanism for excreting toxins and waste from the body.

It is no surprise that when you don't drink enough water, it really does affect your cognition and performance. There are so many people who do not drink enough water every day and are therefore dehydrated. Often, hunger pangs are not signals that you need food, but signals that you are actually thirsty and dehydrated.

Did you know, a human being can survive around a month or more without eating food, but only a week or so without drinking water? Yes, it's THAT important.

By the time you feel thirsty, your body has lost over 1 per cent of its total water. Without further ado, right now is the time to go and grab a big cool glass of the good stuff.

There's this big line here on purpose so you can come back and easily find your place in the book once you've rehydrated.

I know that sounds a bit silly, but it's really easy to forget to drink water. In my work helping people with their own goals and daily discipline, drinking water is the number one thing people struggle with.

GO AND DRINK A GLASS OF WATER

Got a glass of water? Good. Right, where were we? You were here.

With that taken care of, you should know that for men, the average MINIMUM amount of water you should consume a day is 3 litres and for women is 2.2 litres.

Unfortunately, sodas and tea or coffee don't count towards your water intake. Herbal non-caffeinated teas do count towards your total water consumption, and they are a much better alternative than too many caffeinated drinks.

You also may need to up your fluid intake if you live in a hot climate, exercise often or have fever or diarrhoea. Add in an additional 0.5 - 1 litres of water per day if you exercise, even more if you work out longer than an hour.

How to Drink More Water

Firstly, this is one habit that does take a few days to get used to. If you're not currently a regular water drinker, you will find that frequent toilet trips will become quite annoying in the first few days of consuming water regularly. However, I can assure you that this becomes the norm after only a few short days, and the trips will become less frequent.

Many people struggle to drink enough water and to remembering to drink what isn't exactly the most exciting of beverages is the challenge. As the habit of drinking water on a consistent basis is one of the things I find people struggle with the most, here are some tips on how to increase your intake:

Water on waking
As SOON as you wake up in the morning, grab yourself a full pint of water and drink it in one go. You will be dehydrated after sleep, and this is a great way to replenish those fluids.

It will help get your bowels moving. It is also an excellent time to take your morning supplements like a multivitamin, probiotic and Vitamin D if you aren't living somewhere particularly sunny.

Water alarms
Set alarms for water throughout the working day. If you work in an office, this is also a great way to break up your tasks and following the Pomodoro Technique (we will touch on this later in *Step 7 - How to Schedule Like a Boss*) is a great opportunity to stretch your legs and grab a glass.

Carry a bottle of the wet stuff
Invest in a large water bottle and take it with you everywhere. There are even some bottles on the market today that link with your mobile device and can send you handy reminders to drink more water and track your daily intake.

There's an app for that
Track your water intake on a handy app. You could use MyFitnessPal and track your food

there too, or on the iPhone under the Health tab, there is a place to track your water. There are also many apps out there that are inbuilt with regular reminders to ensure you meet your daily water goals.

The return home routine
When you get home from work, make it a habit to set down your bag and keys, take off your shoes and head for a cool glass of water straight away. This will also help you stop picking at food before eating your evening meal and keeping those hunger pangs at bay.

Evening meal
Before your evening meal, enjoy a glass of water. Again, this will not only replenish you but stop you from mistaking thirst for hunger and overeating.

Go herbal
Swap your coffee and teas for herbal non-caffeinated teas that will all go towards your daily water target.

Jazz it up
Jazz up your water - add in fruits such as a squeeze or wedges of lemon, lime, orange and herbs such as mint to infuse more flavours into your water.

2. Make Conscious Food Choices

We human beings love our food. From the moment we are born, we learn that food = love, comfort and the feeling of being satisfied. It is no surprise that we turn to food in adulthood to fill a void and give us a kick and boost.

With our programming, it is ingrained in us to 'treat' and 'reward' with food. But does this really help us? Are the food choices you make with your meals hindering your goal success?

They say that abs are made in the kitchen. Speak to any fitness professional who will confirm that the secret to a magazine-cover physique lies in what you eat, *not* just how hard you train. If your goal is not fitness orientated, it is still relevant as what you eat will fuel your performance and cognition.

Your body spends between 10 and 25 per cent of its total energy on digestion. Foods depleted of natural enzymes take even more energy to break down, leaving you sluggishly exhausted and reaching for that 3 pm pick me up when at your desk.

Think about it. When you eat your Thanksgiving or Christmas dinner, how do you feel afterwards? I bet if you're anything like me you will need to adjust your belt buckle and you'll probably have a little snooze on the sofa within an hour of eating.

In contrast, how do you feel after a mouth-watering fresh salad? I bet the total opposite! The live enzymes in the fresh, uncooked foods help your body break down and digest the food, rather than work against your digestive system.

So with nutrition in mind, it's time to assess what you eat, when you eat and how you eat.

You Are What You Eat

Think about your current nutrition and eating habits. How do your current eating habits affect you? Do you eat for performance? Or are you always in a carb coma?

What do you eat for breakfast? Does it set you up for the day? Or leave you snoozing on the train on the way into work?

What do you grab for lunch? Are you eating on the go? Or maybe not even paying attention to what you eat and munching mindlessly at your desk?

What is for dinner? Are you so exhausted and overwhelmed that you're dialling for the nearest pizza? Or are you meal prepping in advance and coming home to a healthy and nutritious crock-pot dinner?

>>> *Journal* <<<

Using your notebook, take a minute to answer these questions:

- What could I incorporate more of in my diet that makes me feel great?
- What could I eat less of in my diet that doesn't serve me well?

Eating in a Calorie Deficit

All diets work. If followed correctly, all diets will help you lose excess body fat. That is because all diets follow the same principle of helping a person maintain a calorie deficit.

Each one of us will require a certain amount of calories every day made up of four things:

1. Basal Metabolic Rate (BMR). This is the number of calories we need for our bodies to function at rest. Our blood pumping around our system, our brains working, tissue repair, breathing and bodily functions would fall into this BMR category.

2. Exercise Activity Thermogenesis (EAT). This is the number of calories we need for our conscious exercise. That workout we do at the gym, that walk we go on to get our steps up, the bike ride we partake in. Any conscious choice to exercise falls into EAT.

3. Non-Exercise Activity Thermogenesis (NEAT). This is all other movement during a typical day. For example, walking around the house, typing on the keyboard, brushing our teeth, cleaning would fall under NEAT.

4. Thermic Effect of Food (THoF). These are the calories needed to digest the foods we eat.

Each of the above four ways we burn energy is encompassed into one acronym; TDEE (Total Daily Energy Expenditure).

We generate energy through our food and drink (calories), and we need enough energy (calories) for our overall Total Daily Energy Expenditure or TDEE for short.

The calories we need to function at rest (BMR), + the calories from our conscious exercise (EAT), + the calories from all other movement (NEAT), + the calories we need to digest our food (TEoF) = the calories we need each day.

To eat in a calorie deficit, you eat a lower amount of calories than your average TDEE.

To work out your unique calorie intake and calorie deficit requires a number of variable factors like your weight, height and activity levels. Some diets will get you to focus on these specific measurements. Other diets will lead you towards roughly eating in a calorie deficit without being conscious of being in a deficit or even considering calories by using alternative language like points, syns or codes/colour labels for different food groups.

The method of each diet varies. You might follow a points system. You might eliminate whole food groups like a keto diet which removes carbohydrates and therefore a large proportion of calories. You might eat high protein which requires more energy to digest the high protein foods. You might replace calorific meals with shakes. You might adopt intermittent fasting and therefore remove a whole meal out of your usual daily eating regime and therefore remove that calorie intake too. None of these diets are right or wrong. They just all follow the same principle of eating in a calorie deficit.

Eating in a calorie deficit and understanding TDEE was the key for me losing a significant amount of weight and helped cut through the confusion and overwhelm of diet information.

If you would like to delve deeper into the science of fat loss, I have been working with Body Smart Fitness, the online mindset, nutrition and fitness coaching company since 2015. You can find a multitude of science-based resources to help you with your health journey via Body Smart's social media channels **www.instagram.com/bodysmartfitness** or search for the Body Smart Fitness podcast which I co-host.

Finding What Works For You

Many nutritionists advocate a single ingredient food approach because if you've ever embarked on any healthy eating or nutrition change and incorporated more of this into your life, you will have noticed how eating fresh foods help you feel more energised and improve your focus.

However, it's about finding a plan of eating that works for you, what you like to eat and how you live. So whether that's paleo, vegan, ketogenic, a slimming club points method, intermittent fasting etc (the list goes on). Find what works and stick to it. After all the best 'diet' or way of eating is the one that makes you feel vibrant and energised and the diet you can stick to with ease in the long-term.

One question to ask yourself before embarking on any form of diet is to think ahead to the future. Will you realistically be able to do this for the next year, the next decade and the rest of your life? If the answer is no, then it is not a sustainable diet.

For example, if you're hoping that following a low carb, high fat ketogenic diet will help you shift the pounds, but you're looking forward to going back to eating pizza, tacos and burgers once you have got to your goal weight, that isn't something that is sustainable for you in the long term. Unless you work with a professional coach to 'reverse diet' which is a specific process to help you transition back to the way you ate before, while still maintaining your results.

Diets are so personal for each person. I have worked extensively in the diet and fitness industry and can tell you that the people who succeed at losing weight and sustaining results are those who think about weight loss for life, not just to get into that dress in two weeks.

Food Diary

It's time for another little dose of honesty. The only way you can move forward with your nutrition is to assess where you are right now, draw a line in the sand and move on.

Keeping a food diary is a way to visually understand what you are eating and drinking. You can log foods in apps like MyFitnessPal, or you can simply keep a paper record. There are also apps that allow you to take pictures of what you have eaten, presented back to you in a daily gallery. See How You Eat is one of those apps where you can take pictures and keep a visual food diary.

Think back to what you have eaten in the last three days and how you have felt. Using a notepad and pen, make some notes and observations about your food choices over the last few days. Try and answer this with no judgement on yourself. You can't change what has happened, but you can use it as a learning opportunity.

- What did you eat?
- Why did you choose this?
- How did it taste?
- How did you feel after you had eaten it?
- Could you have made a better choice? If so, what was available?

3. Move Your Body

Exercise is the key to physical and mental performance. Participating in a healthy regime which includes exercise you enjoy often creates a ripple effect of positive change in other areas of your life. Exercise can help you feel more energetic, make better food choices, improve your confidence, and improve your body composition. As I mentioned above, it can also help put you in a calorie deficit as you burn calories to fuel your exercise.

Think about how you move your body right now. If you currently regularly participate in sporting activities - good on you! If you don't move your body at present, and particularly if you work in a sedentary role, how can you increase your physical activity for the good of your health and well-being?

Is there an activity that you loved to participate in, as a child, that you could pick up again in adulthood? Did you dance? Do gymnastics? Boxing? Running? There are a multitude of sporting classes out there, and also more gentle and spiritual activities such as yoga or pilates that are effective and challenging.

What could you do for your body? Answer that question, plan in the time and DO IT! I know this is easier said than done but start small, plan in one session a week, get that ticked off and build from there. Even better if you can find a partner to buddy up with and hold yourselves accountable.

4. Look After Your Mental Health

Anxiety and depression are the most common mental health disorders in the UK. According to the mental health charity MIND, 1 in 4 people in the UK will experience a mental health problem each year, and 1 in 6 people will experience a mental health problem such as anxiety or depression in any given week. *[Source: MIND, May 2020]*

Depression and anxiety will not go away with a magic wand, words of encouragement or medication. Depression and anxiety are complex; I am no doctor and not here to play down these serious conditions.

I have been through periods of depression, and I continued to experience anxiety for a number of years. I have sought professional help and coaching for both, and I'm pleased to report that it has been a huge help. I have also made a number of changes to my lifestyle that has had a direct positive impact on my mental health.

Here are some of the strategies I have been encouraged to adopt by clinical professionals. These techniques took a lot of self-discipline to try when I felt low or down, but they truly made a difference. As per the morning routine chapter, I incorporated many of the following techniques into my morning to help shape my mood and internal thoughts for the day ahead.

Meditation

Whether silent or guided, meditation is one of the most effective ways to quiet a worrying mind and help someone to feel empowered to make the right decisions to feel better.

There are apps on the market, including Calm and Headspace which can help you to relax, breathe deep and find the answers within to tackle your worries and problems. Insight Timer is another great meditation app that I recommend for the courses. I find it easy to follow courses for a number of days on different subjects such as anxiety, stress, focus and sleep.

Journal

Recording your thoughts and feelings in a journal, plus the act of actually putting pen to paper can help your mental health tremendously. Instead of having a head full of worries, you can offload your worries in writing and begin to address them.

Deep breathing techniques

Taking a deep intake of breath is extremely calming and keeps you centred. Try it now. Take in a deep breath, hold it for a count of 8 and then breathe out for a count of 8. It will instantly make you feel calmer and in control. If you suffer from anxiety, it is a technique you may have been taught to calm yourself instantly.

Breathe by Dr Belisa Vranich is a well-structured book on breath work. It is a 14-day guide on actively improving the way you breathe.

There's also the Wim Hof Method which is more extreme and also involves freezing cold showers. A few of my friends who work in the fitness industry follow his methods and report that they love it as part of their routine.

Asking for help or reaching out

This was undoubtedly the hardest thing for me to adopt but reaching out to others and being honest about my feelings helped. I have a handful of friends who know my battles with depression and anxiety and being able to seek their advice, words of comfort or just have a friendly and understanding voice on the end of the phone was life-changing.

When I was at my lowest, I didn't want to communicate with anyone, and I would shut myself away for long periods of time. Luckily, I have friends who have been through the same mental health challenges who were able to recognise my behaviour and coax me into talking. The more I talked about it, the easier it became to address how I felt and move on and out of feeling down.

It still takes a lot of effort to ask for help or just someone to talk to. I often feel ashamed when the periods of feeling down hit me, but the more I've reached out, the easier it is to just say "Hey, I'm struggling a bit at the moment, do you fancy a catch-up?" Sitting in my negativity has never been productive and getting out of it by sending that one small message has been so brilliant in getting me back on track.

Asking for help can take a lot of effort. I want to take a moment to remind you that you are outrageously loved by many people in your life. Your loved ones would never want you to suffer in silence. Break that silence with a phone call or catch up and be brave. Speaking out loud about how you honestly feel can be a huge relief.

If you really feel that you cannot speak to your loved ones, friends, colleagues or clinical professionals, many organisations have been set up to provide a listening ear. This short link will take you to the up-to-date list for your country: bit.ly/helplinesbycountry

Treating yourself

In this modern world of hustling and grinding, it is easy to neglect your self-care. Treats, rewards and perks can help cheer you up.

This could be setting aside time for an activity you adore, treating yourself to a massage, a new outfit, that gadget you've had your eye on a relaxing spa day or a night out with friends. Whatever it is, make time to honour and love yourself with some treats.

I find having things to look forward to is very beneficial to keeping those down days at bay. Or even just picking the phone up and chatting to a good friend. Sometimes I will pencil in something as simple as a catch-up as a treat for getting my work done on time.

5. Develop a Strict Sleep Routine

Sleep is so essential and vital to our well-being. Not enough sleep can have a negative impact on your health and well-being, so it is time to implement some rest and recovery strategies.

I can look back on my own journey and realise that getting up early for a morning routine was extremely beneficial. Still, my lack of discipline around going to bed earlier meant I was only getting an average of 4 to 5 hours of sleep per night. I read Matthew Walker's *Why We Sleep* book, which I found hugely inspirational for changing my mindset around the importance of sleep.

I am ashamed to say I used to be someone who would actually say things like "Sleep is for the weak" and "I'll sleep when I'm dead". I think a modern message we see often is 'hustle and grind' and many of us will try and work on a side hustle or a project or business idea that we try and achieve around our day jobs. I often thought that people who slept a lot were lazy, but they are not lazy at all. Sleep is such an integral part of being a human being. Our cells regenerate during rest, and a lack of sleep can cause additional stress on the body.

I thought I functioned better off little sleep as it had been my way of life for a long time. I invested in an Oura ring, a sleep tracking gadget you wear like jewellery. I wear it to bed, and every morning I am presented with my sleep data via the Oura ring app. (I believe that FitBit and other smartwatches and fitness tracking devices like the Whoop band can do the same). Tracking my sleep data started to make sleep a game for me and I wanted to get my scores up, so I adopted methods to get more quality sleep. I began to focus on a strict sleep hygiene routine and am now prioritising getting over 7 hours of sleep per night which is a huge increase for me. My sleep tracking led me to give up alcohol to see if that made an improvement and not only did abstaining increase my sleep quality, but it improved my heart rate during sleep. I have not decided whether I will give up alcohol forever yet, but as I'm actively focusing on improving my sleep at present, I am saying no to it for now.

I am not sure whether it is the additional sleep, the lack of alcohol, meditation or being more active, but I have not suffered from anxiety since making these lifestyle changes.

Your Relationship with Sleep

On average, how much sleep do you get each night at present?

>>> *Journal* <<<

_____ Hours

And how many of the following good sleep habits do you already adopt in your daily routine?

- No caffeine drinks after 4 pm
- Bath before bed
- No electronic equipment 1 hour before bed (TV, PlayStation, iPad, phone, Kindle)
- Journal and empty head of 'to do' list 1 hour before bed
- Light elimination (keeping bedroom dark)
- Hydrate before bed
- Go to bed at a time to get at least 7-9 hours of quality sleep

>>>*Journal*<<<

What will I commit to, to make quality sleep a priority in my life?

A side note on food addiction:

After writing the first draft of this book, I thought about deleting this chapter all together as food is something I had personally struggled with for many years.

In my work as a copywriter, I've written for personal trainers, nutritionists and health coaches for many years. I feel like I have so much stored knowledge of many forms of eating and diets. I've written articles and eBooks on paleo, flexible dieting, IIFYM, ketogenic, veganism, raw foods, low carb, carb cycling, juicing, counting points...the list goes on.

Yet, I felt like a complete fraud writing a book, including chapters on what to eat, when I was stuck in a spiral of compulsive eating and would binge on junk foods at every opportunity. I noticed that I ate my emotions - many people do! I eat when I'm happy, and I eat when I'm sad, and often I don't have the self-discipline to stop.

I knew it had become a problem in my life. After a failed attempt at getting my blood sugar under control with my diet, I came across *Overeaters Anonymous, an organisation linked to Alcoholics Anonymous. I embarked on a program of recovery from my food addiction and attended sessions for a few months. The sessions helped me understand addiction and the emotional reasons underlying my compulsion to eat when times got tough or stressful.

I took what I learned from the sessions and tried to use the awareness I had developed in a way that would allow me a moment to pause before reaching for food. "Do I need this?" "Am I hungry?" "What will eating this do for me right now?" were questions I found myself asking.

I also gained real value from working with an emotional eating specialist called Rachel Foy. Her book, *The Hungry Soul*, is an excellent resource on understanding food addiction and emotional eating. She runs a programme called Soul Fed Woman and has a podcast on the subject of emotional eating.

Eventually, after a lot of work on my mindset around food I realised two really important things that helped me move forwards:

1. I am the product of my repeated decisions (including food decisions).
2. I had held onto a limiting belief that I was a 'terrible' cook for almost three decades.

After reading James Clear's *Atomic Habits* and loving the chapter on taking every goal back to its most basic form, I realised a couple of important truths for me around food. I made a conscious decision to drop the big weight loss goals and food rules I had collected throughout my life. I took it right back to basics and realised that the way that I look is always a product of repeated food decisions over time. It's exceptionally boring and not very sexy but asking myself every day "What decisions do I get to make about food today?" helped a lot.

I started to plan our meals which took the decision fatigue away and those regular moments of staring into the fridge, wondering why I didn't have an appetite for any of the foods there. I had been stuck in a cycle for many years of grocery shopping and buying food with the best intentions of eating healthy, but I was throwing away so much fresh produce every week. That's because I never really had a plan with meals. I'd buy items for the sake of buying them. Cucumbers, for example - oh my word! The amount of cucumbers I have thrown away in my adult life is a disgrace. They always turned to mush at the back of the fridge. I was bulk buying things on offer and not using them within their best before date.

After reading *Atomic Habits* and thinking of my issues with food, I also wondered how I could take the goal of eating healthy back to its smallest action point. If I had realised that not having the right food in the fridge and a plan with food was the issue, then cooking it would be the next action step.

"I'm a crap cook," I thought to myself, and then I had a lightbulb moment that would change everything. "Am I REALLY a crap cook or have I given myself that label?"

I knew it was a label and a limiting belief I had held onto since childhood that I was a "terrible cook". It had all stemmed from one incident and unfortunate mistake. I was 11 years of age, and I had just started high school. It was my second week, and my very first Home Economics cooking class. We were making tomato and basil soup, and I was so excited. The cooking class felt super grown-up, and as my mum was extremely heavily pregnant with my little sister at the time, I relished the thought of stepping up to be the 'big girl' in the family and help with the cooking. I made my fresh tomato soup and cradled it all the way home from school in a flask. My poor mum with her swollen ankles, bad back and enormous bump, shared my pride as she took a sniff of the ruby red contents of the flask. "You put your feet up, mum. I'll warm you some soup up." were my famous last words.

Unfortunately, they hadn't covered reheating said soup in the Home Economics class, so I poured my flask contents and delicious tomato soup into the pretty rosebud patterned ceramic dish and lit the gas on the stove. It was my favourite piece of crockery, and I wanted to present my culinary creation in the best possible way. I carefully lifted the ceramic dish onto the gas cooker's naked flame, took out a wooden spoon from the top drawer and stirred it slowly, taking deep breaths of the fresh, comforting savoury aroma.

BOOM.

Within a couple of minutes, the whole ceramic dish had exploded over the kitchen. The pristine white high gloss kitchen that my mum and dad had worked so hard to afford. It was everywhere—floor, ceiling, tiles, windows and all over me.

That story has followed me around for my whole life. It's the family joke that I am the worst cook. I have said it myself, hundreds or maybe even thousands of times throughout my life. "I can't cook. I am the girl who can explode soup" is the story that always comes out. It was one incident when I was 11, and I did not know better. It was an innocent mistake, and I allowed this intensely humiliating and frightening incident to become true throughout my lifetime.

Once I made the realisation that I had been carrying this limiting belief for so long, I noticed how many times this was presented back to me. My husband is a jokey kind of guy but the number of times he would criticise my cooking or try and take over or just remind me how awful I was at cooking had definitely become a habit for him! At a family meal, I offered my sister some help with the cooking, and she laughed and said: "Nobody wants food poisoning."

This wasn't my family being mean; this was the story I had held onto and allowed everyone to comment on and make true. The truth was I was OK at cooking - when I had a recipe to follow. I invested in some tasty looking recipe books for beginners, bought myself a Slow Cooker Express and started to watch YouTube channels featuring chefs and those passionate about cooking.

I'm sharing this story to remind you that sometimes, we do hold onto limiting beliefs or stories around all sorts of aspects of our lives. I have a friend who identified that she used biscuits as a coping mechanism when she was stressed or upset because she had always been soothed with food as a child. Every scraped knee, tantrum and teary episode had been met with "Here, have a biscuit", and that use of food had continued into her adult life.

When it comes to your health and fitness, there may be limiting beliefs that have shaped your behaviour into adulthood. Maybe you were not picked for the school sports team and have therefore declared that you're "not sporty" as you've grown up.

Maybe you failed at dieting somewhere along the line so in your subconscious you believe "I am a person who cannot lose weight".

Maybe you got injured at some point in your life and have since believed that you can't exercise effectively.

Maybe you were labelled by the way you look at some point in your life, and you have held onto that identity for yourself.

Sometimes, even though we want to change our relationship with food, trying to be super disciplined around what we eat is too hard. We are complex beings with old stories and baggage that we have carried around for decades. We have needed to be nurtured with food and drink since the moment we came into this world, and our individual relationships with food are unique to us and our experiences. Sometimes, taking a moment to look back into your past and assessing whether you have acquired any limiting beliefs or stories around food can help you make more positive choices today and in the future. What did food mean to you growing up? How did it work in your family unit? What foods were used to soothe? What did your parents believe about food? What did you pick up and carry with you that is not your story around food? Answering these questions may help you to unpick the reasons you feel like you don't have discipline with food more effectively than relying on willpower alone.

*If you're reading this and are too struggling with any form of addiction to food, alcohol, drugs, sex, porn, gambling, technology which is affecting your physical or mental health, there is support out there. I encourage you to explore your local 12 step recovery program and attend with an open mind and an open heart.

Step 3

Ways to Stay Accountable

"Accountability breeds response-ability."
- Stephen Covey

While you're more likely to do something and be motivated to do it if you *want* to do it, sometimes you just *have* to knuckle down, be disciplined and get the work done.

After all, overwhelm, and procrastination are two types of FEAR. Procrastination is a person fearing an outcome and responding with the inability to start any action.

Nobody really wants to procrastinate. Nobody wants to feel so overwhelmed that they're stopped dead in their tracks. When these episodes of procrastination come, it is a time to reflect and ask questions:

"Why?"

"Why does this action feel so difficult?"

"What is one small step I can do now to progress me forwards in my goal?"

This is the point where you really do need a healthy dose of accountability to push you along.

So how can you stay accountable?

Staying accountable means taking responsibility for yourself and your daily actions. There are many ways you can be self-accountable, and there are many ways you can involve others.

Could you do any of the following to stay accountable:

Share Your Goals

There's nothing like putting your goals out there to bring them to life. Whether you share them with family and friends, colleagues, social media friends or mentors. Sharing what you want and then stating how you will do it will take that goal from a "here's what I *want* to do" to a "here's what I'm *going* to do" action.

If you just keep your goal in your head, it is easy to drift off from the steps needed to achieve it. It's harder to drift off the path of achieving a goal if you've told those closest to you what you're aiming for and they're asking you questions about it all the time.

Blog About It

Got a blog? Great! Not got one? Why not set one up? They're simple to create on a platform like WordPress, Tumblr, Medium or Blogger, and you can post updates from your phone. You can document your journey as you go along and build a tribe or following as you do.

Make a Video Diary

In the same way a blog is a written diary of your steps towards your goal, a video diary is a way to do it that doesn't require you to write. There are many vloggers out there on YouTube giving a peek and insight into their lives and how they are creating the life they want to live by achieving their goals.

Getting people to subscribe to your journey means they will be notified in their inbox when you post a new video, being able to watch your videos and see how you're progressing.

Join Groups on Facebook or LinkedIn

Depending on your type of goal, there is a Facebook or LinkedIn group for so many different topics.

Want to run a marathon? Join a marathon runners group!

Want to lose 60lb? Join the multitude of fat loss, transformation challenge groups.

Want to improve your pipeline and increase sales by 40% in the next quarter? Again, there will be business groups to help you and offer advice, stay accountable, connect with others and gain valuable insight and information along the way.

Get an Accountability Buddy

For me, this is THE MOST POWERFUL point.

Accountability buddies can work *for you*, or *with you*. By that I mean you can hire someone and they keep you accountable with no responsibility on your part to reciprocate the service, or you can work with someone and have a mutual agreement where you encourage one another along equally.

There are many types of professionals who use accountability as the backbone of their work to help others achieve their goals such as fitness coaches, business mentors and mindset coaches. Then there are communities out there in Facebook groups, or you can get a personal accountability buddy and help one another along.

I have felt really lucky to work with people on different aspects of accountability for different areas in my life.

I have trained 1-2-1 with fitness coaches to learn the correct technique for weight lifting. This type of accountability included weekly check-in calls and reporting to him when I trained outside our sessions (with photographic proof!).

I still meet with my business mentor every couple of months and take an overview of my business performance and plan strategy for the next quarter.

At the point of writing this book, I am working with a mindset coach in a group coaching format. I get the chance to speak with her 1-2-1 a couple of times a month and discuss my personal blocks and what is stopping me from achieving greatness. In the group, we set three weekly actions and report back every Sunday evening on what we have achieved in that week, with proof.

Finally, since 2015 I have had a personal accountability buddy. I've mentioned him before in this book. Ben is an old friend of mine who shares values and goals, and we are there for one another every day. Not only does he do things like call me to get me up, as he lives in a different time zone and is always up when I need to be, but we check in with one another and keep one another on track. We share our action plans for the week and report back with proof that we have completed our agreed actions. In 2019 we also moved all our actions over to Asana project management software, so we really help one another stay on track with our goals and projects.

The above accountability help seems like a lot, doesn't it? But you see, with the exception of my business mentor and working with Ben on my books, all those people help me win at areas of life that are not currently bringing me any income. Areas of life not directly linked to bringing in money are the ones that are the first to get forgotten about in the day-to-day busy madness of running my own business.

I am working on my goals on the side of being a busy business owner and parent. If I didn't have all the support above, I'd go back to playing small and just concentrating on the actions that bring in the money for the mortgage each month.

That's not enough for me. I want to grow. So I have invested in accountability partners to accelerate my journey to my various goals.

An accountability partner can come in the form of a gym buddy, a running partner, a mentor, a colleague who will show you the ropes, a friend or family member. You don't necessarily need to invest any money into staying accountable, but the trick is to find someone who is as dedicated and invested in their goals as you.

Put Your Money Where Your Mouth Is

A great way to stay accountable is to put money on the line. Try handing over some cash to a friend or family member, and you agree to get it back when you achieve different stages of your goal. I talk more about this in Chapter 6, *Sprint v Slow* about the time I paid a stranger £500 until I had completed a specific goal.

If your goal is fitness related, there are apps you can download where you put money into a pot, and earn it back with every gym visit (it is linked to your smartwatch steps and activity and can be GPS tracked so knows where your gym is!). Pact and DietBet apps are two examples.

Put Your Money Where You Don't Want!

On the flip side of earning your money back as above, you could also pledge to donate to a cause that you HATE if you don't complete your actions on time. You would hate that wouldn't you? Donating to something you despise! What a great motivator!

I did this myself in the summer of 2018. I was always late on the school run. My son's teachers had a bit of a word at the end of the school year as my son had been late for school 27 times. That's a lot! And it wasn't his fault, it was mine.

I decided this had to stop, for his sake. So I wrote on my notice board that I would donate £5 every time I was late to the Donkey Sanctuary charity. Why? I really don't like donkeys. A bad donkey ride childhood experience makes me shudder when I think of the creatures. So I said every time I was late, I'd donate it to the Donkey Sanctuary. I was quite amazed at how much this conscious shift worked, and I am sorry to say that the donkeys only got £10 in total from me in the Autumn term.

Sorry donkeys.

Enter a Competition

This doesn't necessarily have to mean a sporting competition. If your goal is to be a writer or world-class photographer, software programmer or chef, there are competitions for every single walk of life.

Entering a competition is a great way to have a final or short-term goal along the journey. Training to win and then the actual competitive nature of your competition means you'll be focused on the prize.

If your main goal isn't related to sporting achievements, it can still be an excellent challenge to enter something like a 5k/10k run, a CrossFit competition, that golfing tournament, or swimming gala to help with your mental and physical performance.

If you own your own business, or your industry has sector-specific awards, why not enter? I do this as part of my day job with my clients, and it is a very rewarding process to reflect on all the positives and achievements of your work or business.

Curb the Electronic Addiction

The modern world is addicted to smartphones and technology. While we have valuable information and content at our fingertips each day, helping us learn at an unprecedented rate, we also suffer at the hands of technology.

If you've ever been super motivated to sit down and begin working on your goal, you've probably experienced the drain and drag of getting sucked into the social media wormhole.

You know what I mean, you've seen a notification pop up on Facebook and the next thing you know you're viewing a myriad of food pictures, baby photos of the girl who you sat next to in Chemistry and your third cousin's recent holiday snaps.

It's just unnecessary and a distraction!

Shutting down electronics while you focus on your goal is such a valuable exercise. In my day-to-day work with clients, the first thing I get any of them to do is to download the Facebook Newsfeed Eradicator Chrome plugin. This means you can access Facebook, see your pages, groups and notifications, but the newsfeed is blank, and instead replaced with an anti-procrastination phrase.

Right now, today's phrase on the Facebook Newsfeed Eradicator is:

> *"Procrastination is like a credit card: it's a lot of fun until you get the bill."*
> - Christopher Parker

Once the news feed eradicator is installed, it's time to think about moving your phone out of reach. Place it on the other side of the room. If it rings, you will hear it and be able to respond.

Turn off your emails, turn off the notifications on any other desktop applications like WhatsApp or Messenger.

Focus your mind and your efforts on your task in hand, and you will be amazed at what you can achieve in what seems like a much shorter time.

If you are worried about the amount of time you spend on social media, you can install apps on your devices that block you from visiting certain apps and sites for different amounts of time. BreakTime is one such app where you can allow yourself allotted times in the day to view social media apps or sites, once your work is done. Moment is another which tracks the time you spend on your devices. It may shock you!

Personally, I found that deleting the Facebook app from my phone was the best thing for me. I noticed I was on Facebook for around three hours a day. That's 21 hours a week. I was losing almost a day of my life each week looking at other people's lives.

I made the decision to try it for a week and see how I felt. With no app icon there on my phone to click onto, I coped. It was strange at first, but I decided to do it another week. And another. I managed 14 weeks without actively accessing my personal profile (I still had to manage accounts for clients), and I realised that I missed nothing.

Because I am not using Facebook as much, I don't have as many notifications. I have also found that I enjoy real-life conversations more. "Did you see it on Facebook?" people will say about their latest holiday or endeavour. It's refreshing to be able to say no, and hear their actual account of things going on in their lives.

Set Up Clear Rewards

Another way to stay self-accountable is to set up mini rewards along the way to your goal. If you have broken down your main goal into actions and know what you're working towards, you can decide and define points along the way as mini-goal markers.

What will you do at these? How will you celebrate? How will you reward yourself?

Regularly Audit Yourself

Auditing yourself and your progress regularly is extremely powerful when it comes to being self-accountable.

In Step 8 - The Weekly Check-in Process we go through this in more detail, but I like to review my progress every Sunday, and I try to do more of an in-depth self-audit on the 1st of every month on my goals and how I am progressing towards the big someday dreams.

I ask myself what went well the previous month and also what didn't go so well. What would I do differently, and how can I improve on this month ahead? I will then usually plan some goals for the month in my journal.

Track Your Progress

Tracking your progress, much like self-auditing, is powerful, so you know where you are at any given time on your goal journey.

If your goal is business or related to finance, you may have a spreadsheet of targets that you fill in and assess each week to notice where you are in your journey.

If your goal is fitness related you may track your sporting achievements; time, reps, personal best stats in a workout journal, or an app like JeFit. You may take progress pictures (highly recommended for anyone with a fat loss or muscle building goal), or you may track your food in an app like MyFitnessPal to stay on the right path to your goal.

Tracking allows you to assess your progress at every stage of the goal journey. If you do this regularly, you can notice areas that need more attention, being honest and realistic about the time you are setting aside for your goal. It can help you see extra steps you may need to implement, extra time you may need to give yourself or extra help you might benefit from reaching out and asking for.

It can be a chore to track, but it definitely helps you to know what you've already achieved and what is next to make your goal a reality.

Journal

I love to track my daily actions and plan them in a journal. Some people do this by blocking time off in their electronic diaries. Others just put pen to paper.

I'm a big fan of the Self Journal daily planner by Best Self Co. The planner features a two-page-a-day spread and gets you to assign half-hour time blocks for all your actions, a space for daily gratitude logs, your main goal and three actions you will take each day and then a space to share your wins and what you learned that day.

It has been one of the most powerful tools in my goal setting armoury, and I can't recommend it enough. Planning out my day, knowing how long things take and being realistic with time and logistics has helped me feel more planned, prepared and ready for each day. It has enabled me to plan realistic deadlines, say no to people when I can clearly see I don't have the time and also realise how long or how little things actually take.

It is wonderful to look back on the Self Journal and see all the action steps I take daily and assess how they are propelling me towards my goals.

Time Track

Much like you can plan out your time in a planner, closely tracking your time when working on a project can be really insightful.

For example, when I started my writing career, I would have a to-do list that was as long as my arm. I would be overwhelmed at the thought of creating four blog posts, a press release and starting an eBook. It would take me days to often get out of the overwhelming fog and make a start.

When I went freelance and started working with multiple clients, I installed an application called PayDirt. It is a time tracking app that not only allowed me to set timers for the different projects I was working on, but I taught it to know which client I was working for, depending on a set of keywords. As I was visiting websites or logging into client websites or Facebook pages of a client, PayDirt would pop up and know which one I was working for, allowing me to start the timer.

Coupled with the Facebook Newsfeed Eradicator and planning out my tasks for the day in my Self Journal, I started to see with a fresh pair of eyes just how long (or how little!) tasks took.

For example, I quickly realised that I could research, write, upload images and publish a 500-word blog post within an hour.

When 'in flow' and writing on a subject I was knowledgeable and passionate about, I could write 1000 words in 25 minutes.

This meant I could complete a 10,000 word eBook within a working day quite easily! It was a shock to realise how little time things took, and time tracking as I went along meant I was less inclined to be distracted by social media, texts or emails. It became a little competition too - me against the timer!

Had I not started time tracking, I don't think I would ever have understood the extent of what I am capable of in a working day. It also allowed me to change the way I work for my clients and see which ones I was over-servicing and which clients needed more time and attention.

I also adopted time tracking at home to help me with self-discipline and my household chores. I am rubbish at cleaning. I hate it because I always wrongly believe it will take me much longer than it actually does.

One day I made a list and timed myself as I went. I now know that the bathroom takes 6 minutes to clean, including scrubbing the bath and shower. It takes 17 seconds to feed my dogs. It takes 2 minutes and 30 seconds to change my bed covers. It takes 48 seconds to take the bin out.

I found once I knew this, I had no excuse, and I stopped putting as many things off. I'm nowhere near as organised and tidy as I'd like to be around the home, but this small activity has helped me see that I have no excuse for not taking an extra 7 seconds to fold a towel or put my shoes away.

Seek Feedback

The last point on staying accountable is to seek feedback from others who have achieved your goal or those who are willing to help.

Sometimes you can put the work in and sweat blood and tears to reach a goal, but if you're doing something wrong, or the long way round, you could be hampering your efforts.

Don't be scared to seek help or feedback from those you admire or look up to. People who have achieved success are generally happy to help others who are looking to better themselves and achieve great things.

Step 4

How to Avoid Goal Overwhelm
The Foolproof Action Plan

"Success is sequential, not simultaneous."
"Focus is a matter of deciding what things you're NOT going to do."
"If you chase two rabbits, you will not catch either one."
                                          - Gary Keller

Firstly, are you overwhelmed? Is this the reason you are reading this book? Are you finding yourself procrastinating even though you know you don't want to be? If so, it sounds like overwhelm! What are the signs of overwhelm, and what can you do to overcome it?

Signs of Overwhelm

- You don't know where to begin, no matter how much you think or try and force yourself to start
- You're not physically or mentally able to start your task in hand
- You procrastinate and do everything BUT the task you've set yourself
- You get headaches or back pain from too much stress
- You forget important things
- You don't find pleasure anymore in the things you used to love

Overwhelm is a horrible sensation that can be caused by overbooking yourself or setting unrealistic deadlines. It can be caused by anxiety or feelings of not being good enough to complete the task in hand. Sometimes, a goal is just too huge and monumental that you don't know where to start breaking it down into smaller, more manageable action steps.

In *Step 7 - How to Schedule Like a Boss*, I talk in more depth about timing things in your life and time blocking. When you time your regular tasks, you will know how long things realistically take you. If you suffer from overwhelm because you over-promise yourself to your colleagues, clients, family, or friends, Step 7 will help you get clear on your most common tasks and set better boundaries for yourself when accepting tasks or actions from others.

When you start to time how long things take you, it means you can plan out your daily schedule with more accuracy. For example, if you know that writing a report takes an average of four hours, you will know to schedule at least four hours into your diary the next time that same task is due. If you know that scheduling social media for your business takes around 10 minutes per post, you can choose to batch create and schedule your content in advance, or you will need to set aside at least 10 minutes each day to post your content.

When you do this often enough with your most regular tasks, you will find yourself plotting out your working week with ease, and the overwhelm should hopefully start to diminish. When you start to get a clear picture of the time you have available, you can confidently say yes or no to further work and responsibilities. You might use this method in the home or at work, for your health or your self-care.

Prioritising Your Workload or Tasks

If you are procrastinating a lot on your day to day tasks, could you redefine the urgency of your daily commitments and tasks? I used to have a system in a former job where we would categorise our daily work into three categories; red, amber and green - like traffic lights. Each morning we would discuss our 'red flag job' as a team and commit to getting that job out of the way first. This would be the job that was proving difficult or was the most urgent. We would hold one another accountable until our 'red flag job' was done and then move onto our amber tasks and so on.

There are many ways to be more efficient with your workload, and if you are serious about getting more done in less time, I highly recommend David Allen's updated *Getting Things Done* (GTD) method and book.

The Domino Effect

Gary Keller founded Keller Williams - a large real estate company, before writing his best selling book, *The One Thing*.

The One Thing teaches you how to have a foolproof daily action plan to ensure your goal actions are consistently moving forwards, much like toppling dominoes, and you're not paralysed by procrastination along the way.

It is a straightforward concept, which makes it such a success, and it has allowed Gary to transform his own life, the lives of his employees at Keller Williams and his global readership who have adopted his One Thing principles.

Straight out of college, Keller began working as a real estate agent and set himself a 'someday' goal of becoming VP of the real estate company he worked for.

He achieved this goal within 4.5 years and focused on it every single day. When he left his original company and founded Keller Williams, he took his own goal setting measures and ingrained them into the company he created, focusing on education of real estate agents and applying his goal principles.

The result at the time of writing this book is that Keller Williams is now the largest real estate company by headcount, and Gary's book has established him as the leader not only in his field but for entrepreneurs as a whole.

So how did he do it? What is *The One Thing*? And how can you follow it too as your foolproof daily action plan towards your goal?

The main idea in the book is based around this one specific question: "What is the one thing I can do such that by doing it, everything else will be easier or unnecessary?"

Read that again a few times. You can use it and apply it in so many areas of life. You can work backwards on everything you're trying to achieve each day and ask yourself which step would be the very first to get your task completed.

In *The One Thing*, Keller also likens this to the power of the domino effect. Every great change starts like falling dominoes.

The following is an excerpt direct from *The One Thing*:

"When you think about success, shoot for the moon. The moon is reachable if you prioritise everything and put all of your energy into accomplishing the most important thing. Getting extraordinary results is all about creating a domino effect in your life.

Toppling dominoes is pretty straightforward. You line them up and tip over the first one. In the real world, though, it's a bit more complicated. The challenge is that life does not line everything up for us and say, "Here's where you should start." Highly successful people know this. So every day they line up their priorities anew, find the lead domino, and work away at it until it falls."

Get the book. It is worth it. Re-read it every year because it will help you stay motivated to achieve those lifetime ambitions.

Start Small and Build Up

Since I first published this very book, I have taken myself and others on a journey of creating small habits at a very basic level and building these habits over time. I encourage people to drill down to the nitty-gritty of the basic tasks and action steps they can take to ensure they're moving towards their ultimate goal.

I go through a specific process with my accountability mentoring clients where we work in 12-week cycles and build on our actions every week. I work with them to get clarity on what their ultimate goal looks like. Then we work backwards and establish the steps or habits that will get them to their goal. We do this because success is sequential. We speak of people as an overnight success which isn't true. Nothing happens instantaneously; success takes hard work and dedication, applying yourself consistently and with focus.

You can speed up success by adopting this principle and know that if you break down your goals into manageable daily actions, you will progress forwards systematically and sequentially, and be more likely to achieve all those things you have your heart set on.

Using Daily Steps In Place of Overwhelming Goals

This chapter aims to tackle overwhelm as it manifests in different scenarios. From daily overwhelm - where your schedule just seems too packed and you don't know where to start to that feeling of overwhelm when a goal feels oppressively huge and you wonder how on earth you will achieve it.

When a goal seems so far out of reach, it can be difficult to get started and topple that first domino.

I experienced this myself with my health goals. As I outlined in the health chapter, after my breakdown, I ate all of my feelings - good and bad! The effect of constant bingeing left my body composition feeling somewhat alien to me. I piled on over 60lbs in a short space of time. It took me four years of continuous yo-yo dieting and trying to be disciplined before I cracked it by focusing on tiny daily actions.

I had always been that big picture person and loved aiming for lofty goals. The idea of losing so much weight felt so big and so difficult. I tried and failed so many times. I'd lose a bit of weight, then put it back on. It was incredibly disheartening, and I know it was not doing my mental health any good. In 2020 I decided to strip every goal I had back to the most basic action. I realised that if I wanted to change my body composition over a certain period of time, that future version of me would just be the result of repeated daily decisions.

I worked out that if I wanted to change in say, 90 days, then I would get to make the following decisions every day:

- Three meal decisions a day
- The decision to drink 2 litres of water
- The decision to move my body and walk 10k steps each day
- The decision to exercise three times per week
- The decision to not drink alcohol (I decided to quit)
- The decision to take my supplements

I then totalled these decisions up and realised that if I wanted to change the way I looked in 90 days, then the person I could become would be:

- 270 meal decisions away from my goal
- 180 litres of water away from my goal
- 900,000 steps away from my goal

- 36 hours of gym sessions away from my goal
- 90 days of no alcohol away from my goal
- 270 supplements away from my goal (multivitamin, omega 3 and probiotic)

I saw that list of the steps broken down and felt like the focus was less on the weight and more on what I could do in the moment each day. "I could do that", I thought to myself.

Life isn't all perfect, and some of those daily action steps were forgotten or missed, but the principle worked. My head went from being terrified of being overweight forever and feeling like the goal was too far out of reach to diligently making positive but small decisions each day.

I even drilled down further and looked at what my domino would be for each of those daily decisions. Meal planning and ordering groceries in advance, having a fresh bottle of water in the fridge, committing with another mum to walk to school, getting my gym kit ready by my bedroom door the night before sessions and having my supplements out ready each night all helped me take each step back to the most basic action and thought. It took away the decision fatigue, and my need for willpower was reduced.

I even used this smallest action step thought process when writing my second book. I initially set a goal of writing 60,000 words in a month. That was broken down to 2,000 words per day. Suddenly, that felt so overwhelming, and I struggled to fit the writing session into my packed schedule. I asked myself what would be the smallest action step in this domino sequence and reframed my daily decision as "I will open my manuscript and place my fingers on the keyboard." Once I took the loaded expectation and meaning I had placed on the word count goal, it felt easy. If I hadn't managed to fit a writing session in, all I needed to do was power up the manuscript document and put my keys on the keyboard. Boom! Daily action step complete! It was so easy to win and tick off that action step every day. I was utterly gobsmacked and furious at myself in equal measure that this method worked so much better for me. There were days when I didn't write a single word and there were days when inspiration would strike as I placed my hands on the keyboard. On one free Saturday I wrote over 10,000 words in one sitting. Would I have done that if I set myself the 2,000 word goal? Maybe not.

Why Does This Approach Work?

This approach of committing to the smallest of action steps works because extraordinary success is sequential, not simultaneous. What starts out linear becomes geometric. You do the right thing, and then you do the next right thing. Over time it adds up, and the geometric potential of success is unleashed. The domino effect applies to the big picture, like your work or business, and it applies to the smallest moment in each day when you're trying to decide what to do next. Success builds on success, and as this happens, over and over, you move toward the highest success possible.

When you see someone who has a lot of knowledge, they learned it over time.

When you see someone who has a lot of skills, they developed them over time.

When you see someone who has done a lot, they accomplished it over time

When you see someone who has a lot of money, they earned it over time.

The key is OVER TIME. Success is built sequentially. It's one thing at a time.

Just like with the geometric progression, when you line up your dominoes correctly, it's the smallest thing that does the most. So when you determine what your first domino is and knock it over, the impact of your action will create a higher level of success.

Apply the Domino Effect in Your Life and Business

Take a look at an aspect of your business/career or life. What's the first domino you need to topple for extraordinary results? In other words, what is the most important thing that will bring the best result in this particular area of life or business and make other things easier or unnecessary?

Define this one thing and focus on that until it is done. Incremental improvements each day will bring amazing results over time.

Remember the question that Gary Keller poses in *The One Thing*: *"What is the one thing I can do such that by doing it, everything else will be easier or unnecessary?"* and apply this principle working down to discover the very first action for each area of your life:

1. Finances
2. Spiritual life

3. Physical health
4. Personal life
5. Business or career goals
6. Relationships
7. Your current job

Exercise: Foolproof Action Plan

\>>> *Journal* <<<

Take the above seven areas of your life and think about your ultimate goal in each area. Take a look at your list and pick the one that feels the most meaningful or important.

Write out your huge goal for that area of your life. Now think about the sequential steps that you might take to achieve that goal. Write them out if you can in a linear fashion. Where do you want to be, and how will you get there? It's easier to work backwards with this way of thinking. Once you feel like you've got to where you are right now with this part of your life, really think deep about the very first tiny action step that you could commit to.

If you feel you have the brain space, and it won't overwhelm you too much, repeat the exercise for each area of your life in the categories above. At the end of this exercise, it is a chance to present before yourself a daily action plan for every area of your life.

Again, remember you can't work on everything at once and depending on the length of time your RIGHT NOW task will take, you may not be able to progress all seven areas of your life in one day.

If you do have the time and are also adopting time blocking methods, you may find that you can do one small action each day in every area of your life that will move you forward - particularly if you are following the Miracle Morning routine. You will find that you DO have more time to plan and implement your daily actions.

Step 5

Getting Out Of Your Own Way

Removing Blocks for a Procrastination-Free Journey

"You gain strength, courage and confidence by every experience in which you really stop to look fear in the face. You are able to say to yourself, 'I have lived through this. I can take the next thing that comes along.' You must do the thing you think you cannot do."

— Eleanor Roosevelt

Let's get serious, and let's get honest.

This is YOUR life.

Not your partner's life, the life of your parents, or the life of your siblings. This is YOUR own life, and it doesn't have to play out like a fantasy movie in your head! There has never been a better time to shape your own life, carve your path and make your success.

Yet not everyone does. Not everyone has the guts, the determination and, of course, the self-discipline to achieve their success.

Why?

The long and short of it is we can often get in our own heads and therefore we create mindset blocks that can get in our way. We create false stories that we allow to define who we are and stop us from progressing forwards.

So what are the most common mindset blocks when it comes to taking action on your goals, and how can you overcome them?

Stop Waiting for the Right Time

There will never be a right time, and your perfectionism is killing your dreams.

It's perfectly fine to dream all these business plans in your head, thinking you will become a global superstar and dreaming of your future desert island and private jet. However, they're no good stuck in your head all day long. Nobody is going to buy an idea in your head.

It's perfectly fine to think "I'll just lose these first 7lbs before signing up to that running club." Do it NOW. There is no time like the present!

We humans sit in front of our computers for hours, days, months and years getting bogged down in unnecessary perfectionism before even launching a beta version of our idea or product and finding out if people will even like or buy it.

A couple of years ago, I went into business with two fitness professionals, and we planned to create an online fitness coaching company. At that time, we were three people with different ideas, values and visions in their heads, all fighting to be heard and create the company.

The first thing we created was the 'perfect' system. We bashed out idea after idea in our heads and knew exactly how we wanted our system to function and operate.

We sought advice from software developers and almost vomited in shock at the five-figure price tag to even get this idea off the ground before we'd secured ONE SINGLE CLIENT.

Yet we went with it. Even though it felt like a massive investment and a huge risk. Before launch, I had a bereavement that became a lot to bear, and I ended up walking away from the business.

I can now reflect and realise that we went about things the wrong way. There was no basic platform that we could upscale along the way – we dive-bombed into perfection, and as such, the idea took well over a year longer and thousands more than it needed to.

The pressure of finances and the differing opinions, coupled with this insane obsession to make everything utterly perfect meant I parted ways with the pair.

The failure on my part in this business taught me some great lessons and mainly the one about being obsessed with perfection. It doesn't exist. Truly. Perfection just does not come into play, and it should never hold you back from starting to work on your goals.

I'm pleased to report that despite the crazy investment, the other two carried on and have created a brilliant and successful platform that helps people all over the world. I still work together within this business, and it's great to see how perfection has been dropped with a focus on consistent daily action across all teams that has enabled the business to thrive and grow by over 400%.

Being successful is about being empowered to speed up the process - not slow it down with impossible perfectionism. Fire it out then tweak. Seek feedback. Learn as you go.

The same with more personal goals. If you want to win that golf tournament, stop fretting about getting into the right club and the right coach, just get down to the driving range and hit a few balls.

When we strive for perfection, is it a reflection of our self-worth issues? If your perfectionism is grinding every plan to a halt, it might be an idea to see a professional mindset coach and reframe those destructive self-worth issues and worry over judgement.

Stop Messing Around on Social Media

I've said this one earlier, and I'll say it again - mainly because I needed to hear it and have truly changed my perspective on this. Facebook, Instagram, Twitter, Pinterest is all just a distraction!

Why do we do it? We can't help ourselves. We sit there with loved ones at dinner, not engaging in conversation, and instead we escape into our devices. WHY?

Why (me included) do we do this? What are we escaping from? Why are we not paying valuable attention and time to those who we love dearly?

It's pretty tragic when you think about it. What will the long-term effect be on our children and the next generation? Are we breeding a tribe of ignorant people who would prefer to busy themselves in an online world than talk to a human being in front of them?

In addition to the worrying effect on our social skills, social media is a time and energy drain. I installed the Momentum app on my phone which tracks how long you spend on your phone each day and then breaks it down into how long you spend on different apps or sites.

When I first installed this app, it was around the time I was suffering from overwhelm and procrastination. I'd just established my own business and felt lost - like I was about to drown. I knew I was spending far too much time on social media and so downloaded the app to tell me just how much time.

This one particular day, the app gave me the news that I had spent 6 hours on my phone looking at Facebook. In one 24 hour period! 6 hours. That is ONE-QUARTER of my whole day!

When you translate that to my lifetime, if I were to live to 80 years old, that would equate to 20 YEARS of my life.

Is Facebook worth robbing me of 20 years? What could I achieve in two decades by putting down the phone?!

Surprise surprise, as soon as this realisation hit me, I worked hard on curbing my social media use. Although it isn't perfect (I work for many clients and curate their social media so sadly have to be on many social platforms) with the news feed eradicator installed on my desktop, it has helped me focus. I also make sure I don't have my phone near me at bedtime and charge it downstairs to remove the temptation of scrolling in bed and staying awake too late.

I also go through periods of time where I can see my social media use creeping up. This is usually due to stress and overwhelm and I find myself endlessly scrolling when I should be focusing on my work. I can identify this behaviour quite quickly now and the easiest instant remedy is to delete the apps from my phone. This might be a temporary measure, say for an afternoon where I am trying to focus, or I might do this for longer periods of time. If I go on vacation with my family I like to turn social media off for the full week and at times I might delete the apps over the course of a weekend to help me stay present with friends and family.

Try it yourself the next time you can feel your life ebbing away to social media scrolling.

Delete your most used social media apps temporarily, and see how you feel about it.

Stop Wasting Your Life on Box Sets

Binge-watching your favourite TV series is definitely one of life's greatest pleasures. It is also sadly one of life's biggest time drains.

My husband loves the TV show Big Brother. Yesterday it flashed on the screen that it was "Day 44 in the Big Brother house".

44 days. One hour of edited footage broadcast each night. I shouted at him:

"How many episodes have you missed of this series."

"Only about three."

Well. You do the math. That's 41 hours of his life that he has wasted in the last 41 days watching a TV show that is watching other people be bored and locked up in a house like some strange psychological experiment.

What could he have achieved in 41 hours? He keeps moaning that his physique is not where he wants it to be. Forty-one hours of work in the gym would've produced some solid results by now.

He always complains that he is exhausted. Well, firstly Big Brother is broadcast late at night, so no surprise there! But if he was exhausted, go to bed an extra hour earlier and get in 41 hours more sleep over the course of just over a month!

Think about how much time you spend watching TV. Whether terrestrial TV, Netflix series or recorded catch up programmes. Are they enhancing your life? If you are a person who watches soap operas, I'd ask you - what do they teach you?

Could you be doing something more realistic, meaningful and worthwhile with your time? Could you be even braver and turn off the TV for a whole week and see how much extra time it gives you?

Go on. Do it. Unplug it. If you do, get in touch and let me know how you found it.

Realise That It's YOUR FAULT

This one is often a bitter pill to swallow.

Not happy with your body shape?

Your fault.

Not happy with your bank balance?

Your fault.

Not happy with your job?

Your fault.

Everything you do in life is a choice. It is YOUR choice. You choose what you get out of this life, and I hope by now after reading all these action steps presented to you, that you could shape your life dramatically if you applied just a few of these principles.

Take Responsibility

Following on from the point above (I know it's harsh and I don't blame you if it's left you feeling triggered) but once you can accept that things are your fault and your choice, you can start to take responsibility and change them.

>>> Journal <<<

I like to advise my clients to do a 'life audit' at this point.

Take every area of your life:

- Finances
- Career/Business
- Love & Relationships
- Body

- Mindset
- Fun & Recreation
- Family
- Personal Growth

With every area, audit it.

- What do you do well?
- What works great?
- What do you dislike?
- What do you attract into your life?
- What could you do more of?
- What could you do less of?

Let's use an example of your career/business. Let's say you work in an office and you hate it. You know you are worth more and can do more. You long to leave your job, or be promoted to another department but at the moment it is a pipe dream.

Answer the questions above about your situation as it is right now. What do you do well in your job, what works great, what do you dislike, what do you want to attract more of when it comes to work, into your life?

Once you've answered those questions, you might decipher what you love about your job or the specific skills you use or the tasks you love. You'll realise what your strengths and weaknesses are.

Next, it's time to TAKE RESPONSIBILITY.

Looking at all the complaints in each area of your life above, know that they are all your choice, and you can also choose to change them.

Let's go back to the career example above. You hate your job. You've established that. You've also established your strengths and the tasks you enjoy.

So how can you take responsibility and reclaim your power here?

Could you take some more courses to sharpen your skills?

Could you be mentored by someone in a position you want - shadow them and gain valuable experience?

If you really want to leave, how will you get yourself noticed? Come up with a job-hunting battle plan. Get your resumé standing out from the rest, get in touch with your professional contacts and scour LinkedIn.

Could you see an opportunity within your company to move sideways or be promoted?

Could you speak up and raise your concerns, demonstrating your case for why things should be done differently?

As you can see, just taking a minute to audit where you're at now, and then take responsibility to change can have dramatic consequences.

I have known many people in my field of work who have experienced a mini-meltdown when it comes to areas of their life, only to accept responsibility and take action. The hardest part is accepting fault; whether with anyone else or yourself, but once you can take responsibility, you can be liberated to write your own script and carve your path with confidence.

Are Your Tribe Your Biggest Block?

Motivational speaker, entrepreneur and author, Jim Rohn, once said: "You are the sum of the five people with whom you spend the most time".

So which five people do you spend the most time with? What do they teach you? How do they make you feel? What are their personal values, work ethic, motivation and drive?

Did you know, if you have an obese friend, you're more likely to become obese yourself! The people around us are huge factors when it comes to our personal success.

Is your partner or your family supportive of you and your dreams? Do they get as excited as you and respect your time to work on your goals? Or do they play the victim and make it all about them when you choose to focus on yourself?

Trust your gut instinct. You are the only person who can write the movie script of your life. You hold the pen and that pen is powerful.

I know it might seem difficult to rewrite your whole life but it is possible. Normal people like you and me quit jobs they hate. Normal people run ultra marathons. Normal people build businesses from their kitchen tables. Normal people get clean of alcohol, drugs or gambling addictions. Normal people uproot their lives and move to new countries. Normal people write books! Every single person who has ever changed the course of their life did so by having the drive to write their new life story and made a series of decisions to make it a reality.

Your new reality might cost you your old one. Which is really hard to think about at times and is another reason we can end up stuck. We grow so used to our comfort zones and our circle of influence that it seems terrifying to break free of that.

You will need to accept the possibility that you're probably going to lose some friends along the way when it comes to achieving your dreams. Some people will get jealous, some will be triggered and you'll make them feel inferior.

That is NOT YOUR PROBLEM.

That is their stuff and if it's causing a problem in your life, it's time to be honest with them and re-establish some boundaries in your friendship. Or if you do find yourselves just not clicking like you used to, it's normal for friendships and acquaintances to run their course. As sad and hard as it may be, sometimes the best thing you can do for yourself, and them, is to let them go.

With other people like your spouse or parents, you're not just going to cut them out of your life, but you can protect yourself by quietly working away at your goals instead of declaring war on anyone who doesn't see and share your excitement for your vision.

It's the reason I love the *Miracle Morning* book by Hal Elrod. You fit your extra work into your mornings at a time when other people are asleep. They don't even need to know about it. You work away diligently, knocking down your dominoes and knowing where you're going.

One day they will wake up and be like "Wow! You got super successful!" Yes. But remember, it didn't happen overnight.

Get Professional Advice from Experts

Another block when achieving your goals might be the fear of failure or not knowing what to do for the best. That's why I am a huge advocate of paying for professional guidance in the form of coaching, mentoring, studying new qualifications or self-studying the works of those who have succeeded in your chosen field.

I hired a social media executive who is 20 years younger than me. Upon offering the role, I struggled to contain my excitement about our future working together. I really enjoy working with young people who are up and coming in their career and it's for one main reason; I don't want them to make the same mistakes that I have made. I want to pass on the last two decades of learning, experience and failure to mould them into the successful person they have the potential to be, in a shorter space of time.

A friend of mine who writes fiction books has just invested an eye-watering sum to be coached by publishing executives so that she knows exactly what to do in order to secure an agent and get a book deal. The shift in her attitude towards this goal has been brilliant and given me goosebumps. She's gone from constantly flapping, stressing and feeling like she'll never achieve this goal to being invested, ready to soak up the knowledge on offer and arm herself with the correct information and guidance to succeed.

Another friend hired a running coach and shaved off 25 minutes on her half marathon time. Something that was really important to her and the definition of goal success.

A woman in my Level Up Facebook group has invested her savings into Neuro Linguistic Programming and hypnotherapy qualifications in order to change her career. She hasn't been happy in her work for a long time, turned 40 and thought "now or never!" so decided to invest the time, energy and money into these qualifications in order to open her hypnotherapy and life coaching business.

When it comes to your goals and achieving them, if you have been stuck it could be time to get the help you need to get unstuck, take action and make progress.

When hiring an expert to help you achieve your goals, do your homework and check. Make sure they have case studies and testimonials. Speak to their past clients and get honest reviews.

Ask plenty of questions otherwise their expert advice could possibly derail your progress.

Getting help might seem like a risk, especially if it means investing a large sum on a consultant, coach, programme or qualification. However, if it is going to save you time, money and energy in the long run, what is that worth to you?

When my friend was accepted onto the book publishing coaching programme she called me to ask my advice. If you've ever agonised over the decision to invest in help or get qualifications to achieve your goals, I'd love for you to ask yourself the same question I asked my friend:

"How much would you pay, right now, to achieve that goal?"

If the answer is more than what the investment of the coaching or qualification is, then work out a way to afford the investment and go for it.

Step 6

Sprint vs Slow

"Your energy is currency. Spend it well. Invest it wisely."
- Unknown

Your energy is not infinite. You do not have unlimited reserves of energy to power you through 20 hour days and unlimited time working on your goal.

If you're going to be efficient in your goal pursuits and achieve your ambitions without burning out, you need to protect your energy, and you need to look after yourself.

Those who choose to go down this self-discipline path and achieve great things often make a short-term sacrifice. We all know that goals and dreams take time. Sometimes, you can be a busy fool and leave yourself no extra energy to truly focus on your ONE THING and get your actions completed.

In this step, I encourage you to tune into your mindset and your body and learn to read yourself, to understand when to sprint and when to slow down.

During the industrial revolution, when factories relied on employees working in shifts to keep the production line going, it was the norm to work 10-16 hours a day. Men, women and children all put in the hours to complete the work and get paid.

Several union guidelines, international government papers and books were published in the late 19th century encouraging a change to working hours. Still, it was Henry Ford who became the pioneer and the father of the 8 hour working day in the early 20th century.

He promised to let his workers work 8 hours a day, for five days a week while guaranteeing the equivalent of six days pay. Productivity increased, and this small change resulted in huge profits and results for Ford.

However, this was over 100 years ago when the world was completely different.

Our working environments are experiencing a contemporary overhaul. Look at giant companies like Google, Facebook and Tesla and look into their working practices. They implement benefits, perks and create working environments for us as we live and work *today*. Ford implemented his 8 hour day and five day week because it was the right thing for the time. So what is the right thing for this modern time?

We do things so much faster and better with the advances in technology. Many forward-thinking companies of today are adopting measures for the modern-day workforce like working from home, flexi-time, and meetings done via video link rather than international travel. We work smarter, not necessarily longer.

Yet, as I write this, I know that I can work longer and it will benefit me. I am trying to cram in as much work as possible before the summer holidays. As a parent, my childcare options become limited over the summer. It has meant that I have been working early every morning before my son wakes, and then again in the evening when he has gone to bed. My days are a mixture of child-friendly activities bookended by the work I need to complete to get paid.

What a luxury! Being self-employed means I can do this. If I worked the equivalent of an 18 hour day in an office, I think I'd get fed up with it and feel drained. It isn't for everyone, but this is a perfect balance for me in that I spend quality time with my son whilst also working on my business. It causes a shift in mindset and feels like a privilege rather than a curse – I get the best of both worlds.

I'm also limited in time in the mornings and evenings, so I find I naturally work quicker and smarter. I have to get tasks completed before my son wakes, so I am constantly working to self-imposed deadlines.

This is also known as Parkinson's law. Parkinson's law is the adage that 'work expands to fill the time available for its completion.' Or alternatively phrased as 'the amount of time which one has to perform a task is the amount of time it will take to complete the task.' So in a nutshell, choosing to cram my work into shorter time frames actually works to the rules of Parkinson's law and I find I do get it all done, most of the time while trying to be a good mum.

I also know I can't do this long-term—maybe four or five days maximum before I crash. I'm into day three at the moment and have planned a chilled out afternoon, knowing I need to top up the energy reserves later.

I'm not writing this to suggest that you should in any way follow suit. I'm just pointing out that a 9-5 pm role, 40 hours a week doesn't have to be the norm, nor does it have to get in the way of you achieving your goals outside of your job.

There are 168 hours in each week, and if you're working 40 of them and sleeping for 56 of them what are you doing for the other 72 hours in a week? And could you dedicate some of those hours to self-disciplined actions that will, in turn, lead to great habits and feeling happier and in more control of your life?

Paying £500 to a Stranger to Sprint

Another way you could push yourself to sprint through your goal is to participate in an organised sprint. I am part of Atomic - the online business club created by Andrew Pickering and Pete Gartland (professionally known as 'Andrew and Pete'). Atomic is a Facebook group, website and series of online events designed for small business owners to upskill and uplevel their businesses. Part of the calendar of activities is a two or three week organised 'sprint'. You commit to specific tasks and outcomes that you will be able to perform in the allotted time frame and place a wager. If you can prove (with concrete evidence!) that you've completed all of your tasks you get your money back. If you fail at your sprint, you lose your money and it goes on the bar tab at Andrew and Pete's annual Atomicon conference.

The first time I participated in the sprint process with Atomic I didn't know anyone personally, had never met anyone and I was handing over cash (albeit via Paypal) to strangers. The first time I did the sprint process I committed to so much! But the thought of losing my £500 wager made me super conservative with my time and I got all my evidence submitted 10 minutes before the deadline! I completed my actions, got my refund and was really shocked at how much I had managed to achieve when the pressure and stress of possibly losing so much money was on my shoulders.

I have also done this with 90 day accountability challenges I have organised with friends. We committed to specific outcome goals and daily processes for a 90 day period and each made another £500 wager. This time it was health and fitness related for me and in the 90 day period I achieved my weight loss targets, got my money back and promptly invested it into some well-earned new clothes.

Jo Macfarlane's 5-9 9-5 5-9 Method™

Jo Macfarlane is an award winning candlemaker, small business mentor and author of *Ask and Act*. She's also a really good friend of mine and someone who I class as a kindred spirit. Jo works super hard to fit in all her goals into her life. I do class her as a real life super woman as she's either parenting, candle making, committing to reading 100 books in a year or doing some gruelling sporting challenge like running the length of Britain or winter sea swimming!

Jo has a method that she adopts when working on a specific goal. She calls it the 5-9 9-5 5-9 Method™. This is essentially working 5-9am on your goal, working at your job 9-5pm and working on your goal again 5-9pm. Now she's not super rigid with these times and she still has responsibilities or self-care activities like exercise, cooking and household chores to do. She doesn't indulge in TV at this time, curbs her social media use and is strict with her time management. Jo is a fellow lover of *The Miracle Morning* by Hal Elrod and has adopted his method of SAVERS to help her commit to her many personal and business goals. It might sound extreme working from 5am to 9pm but it's not forever, it's for a short period of necessary growth where she likes the feeling of working hard on her next project. Jo sets herself a few days or weeks of following this method until her goals are complete. She doesn't do this year round, but she commits to this method of working when she has a business project to finish, like when she created her hugely successful online candle making course.

I'm not suggesting that you should be working 16 hours a day but if you are serious about achieving anything in your life that means something to you, start to assign times when you will work on your actions. Time banding when she can and can't work on her goal helped Jo and it could help you too. Even an hour a day would mean 365 hours a year or the equivalent of just over 15 days. What could you achieve with 15 extra days a year?

When Are You in Flow?

Being able to sprint involves being in flow. What is flow?

Also known as 'being in the zone', being in flow is a term coined in positive psychology when your mental state of operation is at its optimum level. It's when you're fully immersed in an activity where you're fully focused, feeling energised, experiencing full involvement and enjoyment in the activity. You're completely absorbed in your action, and you're losing the sense of space and time.

Have you ever experienced being in flow? If so, what were the circumstances around it? How could you replicate that for the times you're looking to sprint and get stuff done?

I recently had the use of a recording studio for a couple of days while recording the audio-book version of this book. This studio was soundproofed and had no windows. I spent 18 hours there in total, drafting and amending chapters along with recording sections of the book. I loved every single minute of it. I arrived at 9 am and left at 3 am, and it felt like I'd been there for about 4 hours. The next day I was expecting to be tired, but weirdly I wasn't.

I think the absence of windows and clocks had tricked my mind completely. I had no concept of time and was just focused on getting my work done, enjoying it in the process. I've since worked from studios with no windows and clocks and loved it, once again tricking my mind on the concept of time. I have realised that this is my sweet spot and the perfect environment when I want to get my head down and achieve goals in a short space of time, in one sprint. This is the right environment for me to be in flow.

I also know that even when nobody else is home with me, working from home rarely helps me be in flow unless it is early in the morning and quiet. So if I have to do focused work that requires a sprint, I try and take myself away from home.

I have booked AirBnB properties or hotel rooms for myself a few times when it came to finishing writing projects that I couldn't seem to complete. My friend Laura and I booked a quaint little cottage in Yorkshire and took ourselves away for a girly working holiday. We wrote and created so much over the course of a few days and want to make this a regular business break.

I also make use of shared co-working spaces where you pay to use the facilities. I am a big believer in energy and vibes from others, and I love going to these shared working spaces in the city centre, feeding off the energy of other busy working people using the space.

When Do You Need to Slow?

It's all very well focusing on the need for speed in life and work, but it's equally important to slow.

If you were a regular gym-goer, your trainer would always emphasise the importance of a rest day. You can't keep your foot on the gas and slowing down is equally as important as speeding up.

Planning in times to slow down can also act as a reward and drive you to achieve your goals in your sprint periods. If you know you have some downtime planned in, use it to fuel you to get finished.

A friend of mine who owns his own business and tends to work away a lot makes sure he plans one evening a week for a digital detox. No phones, no TV, no computers, no tablets. It's the same rule for his whole family, and they make sure they do something worthwhile and spend quality time together with no distractions.

Sprint v slow is all about balance, and you need to figure out the best way to make it work for you.

Dan Meredith, the author of *How To Be F*cking Awesome* documents his own sprint and slow methods on his Coffee with Dan Facebook groups and his process is fascinating.

He works in 90 day sprints and then 90 days of working at a slower pace.

In a 90 day period, it's all work work work. He writes books in a matter of days, creates brand new online programmes overnight and launches new businesses.

Then, when 90 days are over, it's time to slow. Dan uses this time to still work on his businesses, but he tries to use this time to focus on fun and travel. Check out one of his many posts and videos of him playing on his jet ski, or taking himself off to a foreign city for the day. Honestly, the guy is ace and worth a follow if you don't already. Search 'Coffee with Dan' on Facebook.

Theming Your Days

Jack Dorsey, the CEO of Square and one of the founders of Twitter, is the champ of sprinting.

He worked 8 hours a day for both companies at the SAME TIME for a while when Square was being established. He said, "The only way to do this is to be very disciplined and very productive." He didn't do it forever, eight months I believe, but he was strict about having the weekends off completely, and he also structured his working week by theming each day.

Jack Dorsey's days looked like this:

Monday: . . . . Management meetings

Tuesday: . . . . Product

Wednesday: . . . . Marketing, comms and growth

Thursday: . . . . Developers and partnerships

Friday: . . . . Company structure and recruiting

Having this structure meant he always knew that if a task cropped up to do with marketing, for example, he'd deal with it on a Wednesday. He was able to stay focused and work this way for an extended period.

If you're self-employed and have flexibility with the way you structure your work, many entrepreneurs recommend the sprint method for the start of your working week.

If you can figure out your most important and time-consuming tasks you do week in, week out, try to get those done at the start of the week, working late if you have to (this is what a few entrepreneurs I admire do). That leaves the rest of the week for creativity, growth ideas, and actually working ON your business rather than stuck IN it. Or even better, it leaves you with the time to rest, relax, learn or be creative.

If you don't own your own business and your goal is to be more organised in the home, better at work, or a health or fitness goal, could you adopt the same thinking? Could you challenge yourself to pick up the pace at the start of the week and complete those tasks leaving you with a bit of thinking and wiggle room for the latter end into the weekend?

Working Out Your Sprint v Slow Limits

Do you know your own Sprint v Slow limits?

Do you know how much you can take on and the point at which you really need to slow it all down?

Do you know your weekly non-negotiable tasks in your life and business that MUST be completed? The tasks that you could maybe look to start completing at the start of the week, freeing up time later in the week for those slower days?

Have you been pushing too hard and over-training? Are you giving your body the rest it needs? Are you eating enough ahead of that sporting competition, to give you the edge?

When was the last time you went on holiday and truly switched off? We are so connected to our devices these days that it has almost become the norm to still be in contact with the office when we are away, which never fully allows our brains and bodies the chance to rest and recover.

So, if you are feeling the burn of burn out and know that a slow down process is well overdue, could your ONE THING today be to do just that for yourself?

A massage, a 10-minute meditation, a chat over a cup of coffee with a good friend, a relaxing steam and sauna session at the gym, your favourite meal out for dinner? What could you do that will help you slow?

Are You Really Tired Though?

One thing that stops me from being in 'flow' and being able to sprint is not actual tiredness but perceived and false tiredness.

Try this exercise out for size today:

In the course of your day today, notice how many times people say "I'm tired" or a variation of it:

"I'm shattered."

"knackered."

"I'm done in."

"I'm exhausted."

I think you will be shocked! I believe that we say this out of habit, rather than listening to our bodies and assessing how we feel.

"I'm sick and tired of always being sick and tired!"

Another great exercise is for anyone who is sick and tired of always being sick and tired. For a week, try and STOP saying that you are tired. I did this and was shocked how much I said it, and how it then made me feel, well, tired!

Just like someone yawning in front of you will make your mouth and throat twitch into the yawning action, saying you are tired makes you feel tired. I'd encourage you to ask yourself the question "Yes, but am I really?".

If you aren't actually tired, well then you've got more time and energy to dedicate towards your goals.

Step 7

How to Schedule Like a Boss

"There are dreamers and there are planners; the planners make their dreams come true."
- Edwin Louis Cole

It was Benjamin Franklin who wrote "Time is money" to convey the monetary cost of laziness, procrastination and inefficiency.

If you happen to work on a fast-paced production line, you know that every second is accounted for. Much like the Sprint vs Slow theory in the previous chapter, there is zero time for chatter and distraction on a production line.

You work to your absolute limit and best, diligently completing your tasks, and if you mess up, the whole production line stops. It is a huge responsibility, but proof that focusing on your task in hand with zero distractions gets the job done!

It's time to apply that principle to your own life.

Have you ever heard of a Pomodoro timer and the Pomodoro technique?

The Pomodoro Technique is a simple time management system developed by Francesco Cirillo in the late 1980s. Remember the old style tomato timers you would have in the kitchen in the 80s? Use one of these mechanical timers to break down your tasks into 25-minute segments, separated by 5-minute breaks.

These breaks or intervals are named Pomodoros, the plural in English of the Italian word pomodoro (tomato), after the tomato-shaped kitchen timer that Cirillo used as a university student.

There are six steps in the technique:

1. Decide on the task to be done
2. Set the Pomodoro timer (traditionally to 25 minutes)
3. Work on the task until the timer rings
4. After the timer rings out, put a checkmark on a piece of paper
5. If you have fewer than four checkmarks, take a short break (3–5 minutes), then go to step 2
6. After four Pomodoros, take a longer break (15–30 minutes), reset your checkmark count to zero, then go to step 1

Or suppose you are a person who works in a busy place with lots of distractions, or you need to speak with colleagues regularly to complete your work. In that case, you can choose to set the Pomodoro timer to 25 minutes and use the 5-minute break in between each one to touch base with your colleagues.

If you are interrupted during a Pomodoro, you are encouraged to pause the timer and resume when you are distraction-free.

There are apps that you can download to your phone or desktop which incorporate the Pomodoro method, and allow you to track tasks completed and time taken. I have used this method myself for the last few years and found it particularly useful in my previous corporate role in a busy office.

If you do find yourself in a busy office getting distracted by colleague chatter, then try wearing headphones. Even if you have no sound coming through them, you'll be shocked at how it helps people stop disturbing you.

My FREE Pomodoro inspired 60 Minute Guided Focus Audio

I created a 60 Minute Guided Focus Audio track that has been inspired by the Pomodoro Technique.

The 60-minute focus track features a short meditation at the start to ground you and set you in the right frame of mind to kick procrastination for good. Once the short meditation is over, you will be guided through two Pomodoros and two breaks. I have specially selected very relaxing music complete with binaural beats for maximum concentration.

To get your hands on a FREE copy of the 60 Minute Guided Focus Audio, please go to: **www.gemmaray.com/pomodoro**, and you will receive it by email.

The Sunday Night Weekly Spread

Many people like to plan their week ahead and feel in control of their schedule. Where possible, I like to assign 30 mins every Sunday afternoon or evening to plan my week ahead. I use a planner that is broken into days of the week, hour by hour, and I like to plot what is happening in advance each Sunday. I fill in the family stuff first and the non-negotiables (son's football training, the family party, the mandatory meeting on a Thursday morning etc). I try to add in the places where it's likely there's enough time to exercise. Then I go back over my emails from the week before, go back through my Self Journal at the tasks still in hand and I make a list of all the stuff that is required of me that coming week. I'll also look at the calendar for the upcoming week and I've even been known to run a search on WhatsApp or Messenger messages for dates or days of the week to see if I've made arrangements in the moment that may not have been noted in the calendar. Using all the info at hand, I'll look to see what needs to get done? Are there any strict deadlines? Am I waiting on anyone else to complete my parts of certain upcoming tasks? Who do I need to nudge?

I have also got into the habit of using the Best Self Co Weekly Action Plan for this. Best Self Co is the creator of the Self Journal. Their productivity products are world-class for getting your life in order. I will look at my to-do list in all areas of life; work, clients, personal, family, home and just write down everything that needs to be done on the Best Self Co Action Plan pad. I fill in the estimated time needed for each task, the due date and the priority so I can then cross reference with my own upcoming weekly spread and start to plot in realistic times so I can get things completed.

Reading this back, it all sounds more overwhelming than it actually is. It takes a bit of time getting used to cross-referencing everything – particularly if you're in demand from many different people and projects in any given week. Doing it this way and having the master to-do list and the weekly spread allows me to see everything that is expected of me at a glance. It gives me a 360-degree view of the expectations placed on me and helps me get clarity on what I can delegate or what is not actually that important. It allows me to prioritise tasks, but most importantly it allows me to prioritise me and my own needs first.

A couple of great questions you can ask yourself when planning your week ahead:

"Is this important?"

"Is this important right now?"

"Is this something I need to do?"

"Who else could do this or help me complete it?"

The "Is this important RIGHT NOW?" question is usually the most thought-provoking and gets you to realise what really is the priority in your week ahead.

My friend Stacey has a good way of visualising this when a to-do list gets a little overwhelming. Think of all your tasks as juggling balls. While you might be doing your best to keep them all up in the air, ask yourself which of your to-do list juggling balls are made of plastic and which are made of glass? When I visualised this myself I found it really helped me prioritise the necessity and urgency of those tasks I would label as 'glass' when thinking of them as juggling balls.

The Self Journal

I have already mentioned this in Step 1 and above, but I am a big fan of the Self Journal by Best Self Co for breaking down time blocks every morning and knowing what you will work on.

A simple paper diary and tracker, the Self Journal was born after the developers interviewed the world's leading entrepreneurs to find out their secrets of success.

Scheduling tasks, gratitude, focusing on goals and sharing wins and lessons learned became the backbone of the Self Journal, and I have to say, it has been one of the most powerful tools I have used since deciding to change my life and focus on my goals.

Other Time Blocking Apps

Plan
Plan is simple and powerful and looks great with a clean user interface. It's part to-do list, part calendar, and all business plus loads of extra features that quickly set up blocks of time for priority tasks and projects.

Plan is very much like a shopping or to-do list app but with a twist. The app shows your Google Calendar side-by-side with your to-do list, so you can drag-and-drop tasks into your calendar. (You decide whether or not others can see these focus blocks on your calendar.)

It also includes Day/Week/Month view options, as well as the ability to create lists and projects to further organise your tasks. Plan also gives you data including the average time spent on a task or offers insights into key activities like taking lunch or exercising (by pulling keywords like 'walk' or 'lunch' from your calendar appointments).

Google Calendar/iCal
Whether you have an iPhone or Android, the in-built calendar is a brilliant option for time blocking. As with all-time blocking planning, it is advised to decide on the time you will take on tasks first thing in the morning when planning your day and looking through your actions.

Your calendar can be broken down into 15-minute increments, but you can colour code and add invitees, alerts and notes to your calendars to ensure that you are super-efficient with your time blocking.

Don't forget to schedule in the stuff for you. Don't make it all about work work work. If your goal is to do with your body composition or sporting achievement, make sure you put appointments with yourself in the diary. That way, you will be more likely to stick with your training, your meal prepping or your stretching, for example.

PayDirt
On the flip side, if your job or goal in hand is more reactive than proactive and you're still looking for a method to see how much time a task has taken, I highly recommend PayDirt.

You pay a monthly fee to use it, but not only does it know what you're working on thanks to predetermined keywords, but it time tracks AND creates invoices which can be paid directly into PayDirt via PayPal or Stripe. Pretty cool, eh?

Pitfalls with Time Blocking

When you first start to time block your tasks, you will be tempted to cram in too much and not be realistic about how long things take. This is completely normal.

When first beginning to time block, start small, with a couple of tasks. Decide on two tasks that you complete regularly and schedule a time in the morning and a time in the afternoon to complete these.

Follow all the other hints and tips in the book to avoid distraction like utilising the Facebook Newsfeed Eradicator, turn off emails, turn off your phone and deep dive into your tasks at hand.

Work ONLY and solely on that task. Once complete, notice how long it took you. Make a note of it and know that this task generally takes [x] minutes. This will come in handy in the future when you are time blocking.

It takes a couple of weeks to get used to the process of assessing how much time you will need for all your tasks. Once you are in the swing of it, you will wonder how you ever got so little done in the past!

Two Minute Tasks – Do It, It's Done!

There will be many tasks you complete in your day to day life that don't really take much time at all.

If you have regular tasks in your life that take two minutes or less, the rule of thumb is "Do it, it's done!" (thanks to my friend Kerri for that one). It's also one of the easiest lessons in David Allen's *Getting Things Done* book, where he stresses the importance of tackling 2-minute tasks as soon as they crop up.

When I started time tracking, I also started time tracking chores and tasks in the home and was shocked at how little time some of them took.

Then, when I started using the Pomodoro technique, I found I used my 5-minute breaks to walk around, and I might do a couple of these 2-minute tasks.

I kept a little note of how long things took. My 2-minute tasks are ridiculous, but I always put them off. Here's some of mine:

Make my bed: . . . . 30 seconds

Feed the dogs: . . . . 17 seconds

Take out the bin: . . . . 48 seconds

Change the loo roll: . . . . 7 seconds

Put the dishes away: . . . . 2 minutes

Put a load of washing on: . . . . 1 minute 45 seconds

Put a load of washing in the tumble dryer: . . . . 50 seconds

Text my husband: . . . . 25 seconds

I remember looking at my list and laughing at the absurdity of it all. Why had I continued to think these small tasks were better saved for later?

Now I think "Do it, it's done!" in my head and I get it done. It still doesn't come easy, and my natural default behaviour is to want to put it off, but when I do it and get it done, it really does leave lots more room up in my head for other tasks and I do get a bit of a buzz ticking these small tasks off the list.

Step 8

The Weekly Check-in Process
Monitor Your Progress Every Step of the Way

"Today's progress was yesterday's plan."
- Unknown

You've set a goal, and you're going to achieve it! You're motivated and excited, and you can't wait to get started.

Maintaining that momentum is the hardest part of achieving any goal. Monitoring and tracking your progress are the things that will help you maintain that momentum.

The art of tracking your goals is a self-discipline action in itself. If you don't monitor your progress, you won't know if you're moving in the right direction and it's easy for those action steps to slip out of sight.

Tracking your actions helps you focus.

Between 2016 and 2018 I gained 60lb in weight. I can guarantee if I'd tracked my progress every week, asking myself honest questions about my behaviour around food and exercise I probably could have staged my own intervention. Alas, I didn't. My focus shifted onto my own business, I quit the gym, and the weight crept on rapidly.

Now, this weight gain and noticeable change in appearance was actually a worthwhile experience as it taught me that I am someone who goes off the rails with food and makes excuses about exercise if I'm not tracking or being held accountable.

When I finally jumped back into tracking my nutrition and exercise, I immediately felt more mentally focused and clear – noticing correlations with my food choices and moving my body with having more energy and feeling better all round. Tracking my food helped me stay in a consistent calorie deficit and lose the excess weight.

Tracking my food in advance of eating it turned out to be the secret to my eventual weight loss. Planning meals in advance reduced stress and I was able to be more organised with shopping. Tracking what I would eat each day in the morning, before I ate it, ensured I stayed within my calorie and macro goals. Of course, it wasn't perfect every day but planning in advance took away the decision fatigue and need for willpower which I think is why I love planning so much. Planning creates valuable mental space.

The Sunday Self Audit

The Sunday Self Audit is inspired by Lewis Howes from The School of Greatness, who does admit that he doesn't get this right every week, but when he does it's worthwhile.

The idea is that you use time each Sunday to look back at the week that has just passed and audit yourself. Then once you have a baseline of your week just gone, you can plan your week ahead.

I don't know about you, but when I was employed in my full-time job, every Sunday night I'd get 'the fear'. That flutter in your tummy anxiety for the week ahead where you'd think "Oh god what have I not done last week?" and "Oh crap, what have I got coming up this week?"

That's why I love the Sunday night self-audit. It lays out everything on the table and helps me look at my upcoming week in a proactive, rather than reactive manner.

Every Sunday set aside some time, as much time as you can allow. As explained in the previous step, I like to take around 30 minutes to plan my week ahead in my weekly planner. This self-reflection back across the past week forms the first part of that Sunday planning session. It only takes around 10 minutes, but if you've got time for an hour, even better!

The point is to look back over the week and ask yourself some really important self-audit questions. Here are a few examples for your reference. You might choose to ask yourself the same questions every week, you might choose to answer a mixture, you might choose to put pen to paper with no expectations and write down how you truly feel.

Example self-audit questions:

- What are my goals?
- What was my intention for last week?
- How many of my tasks did I complete?
- What was the best thing that happened/greatest win?
- What lessons did I learn?
- How much further am I towards my someday goal?
- What else could I do this week?
- Which areas of the week did I perform best?
- Which areas were a challenge?
- What is important now that wasn't before?

Once you've asked yourselves these questions, work out the plan for the week ahead.

- How much free time do I have this week?
- Where do I need to focus?
- What are my three main intentions for the week ahead?

Once you have reflected on the week that was, it's time to plot the week ahead. As explained in the previous chapter. Yes, I know it sounds like a right pain in the backside doing this but trust me, you feel so much calmer going into Monday knowing exactly what you've got coming up.

Group Self-Audit

I've been part of mastermind groups where many people complete these kinds of exercises and report back every week. This was always the most beneficial way for me, because I knew I had a deadline and I knew I'd get kicked out of the very supportive group if I didn't do my Sunday assessment!

This is exactly why I chose to create and run my own dedicated 90 Days to Change Your Life programme. I have been part of so many different masterminds that I feel I know the right formula for creating one that really keeps people motivated and entertained at the same time. After all, if it's not fun then you won't stick to it!

My 90 Day Programme has a set structure with members able to 'check in' with their weekly progress between Friday evening and Sunday evening. The group offers support and feedback, as do I, and we constantly help one another progress forwards.

To enrol or find out availability on the next 90 day programme, visit gemmaray.com.

Different Ways of Tracking

Benjamin Franklin famously tracked his progress every day in 13 week cycles and asked his probing question each night; "What good have I done today?"

You don't necessarily need to track your progress daily, weekly is often enough.

The Wheel of Life

One method you could use each week, which is visual and powerful is The Wheel of Life.

The Wheel of Life can be drawn easily in any journal. Draw a circle and split it into 8 different sections and fill it in to give you a score out of 10 in each area:

- Finances
- Personal Growth
- Health
- Family
- Relationships
- Social Life

- Attitude
- Career

Ask yourself where you are right now in every area of your life. With 10 being the best and 0 being the worst.

I use the attitude section of the wheel to describe my attitude to my goals and my general motivation to achieve them.

When you complete this exercise regularly, you start to notice patterns emerging and you can see which areas need more attention to bring up the score.

Tracking Spreadsheet

As described in the accountability chapter, using a tracking spreadsheet is another great way of seeing your progress written down each week.

It doesn't have to be anything complicated or fancy as it will be for yourself and possibly your accountability buddy or mentor to look over together and assess. You can use an online system like Google Sheets to be able to access it on the go, or share with an accountability buddy or mentor.

Keeping track is the very best way to not let things slip. It doesn't need to take lots of time either, a simple tracking spreadsheet can be set up within an hour.

Tracking Apps

There are some great habit building apps out there where you can 'collect' each positive habit or action completed in order to get a streak of ticks or marks on your progress chart.

A few apps on the market at the moment that are great for this include:

Productive – Habit Tracker
Available on iOS for iPhone and iPad, Productive lets you set your own habits and actions in different categories and also set them in different day parts, days of the week, weekly or monthly. It will even send you reminders! For example, there is a reminder that goes off in the morning, afternoon and evening which reminds you to check your posture. If you complete

the habit, you check the box and build up your habits gaining access to further levels.

Habit Bull – Habit Tracking App

Habit Bull is available on both iOS and Android. It's one of the nicest interfaces for a habit tracking app with colour coded date rings that make you want to tick off your habits to keep it looking so pretty. The free version allows you to track up to 5 habits and it has no ads, even the free version. The paid version includes reminders, being able to export your own data, widgets for Android, in-depth analysis tools, multi device syncing and access to the Habit Bull community where you can share habits and ideas.

Habitify

This is really clean and elegant in design and also includes a handy digital journal function. Habitify also produces graphs and data about your daily routines to help you see your week at a glance and where you might need to reallocate more time and effort.

HabitShare

This habit sharing app allows you to track your habits with friends or family for extra accountability. You can have total control over privacy and choose to share certain habits with people or keep them private to just you. You can message friends in the app and keep them motivated with gifs and emojis. Features include reminders, streaks, charts, daily and weekly habit goals, sync across devices and flexible habit schedules.

Fabulous

This is my app of choice and it's so good I paid for the annual membership. Developed by behavioral psychologists, the app gets you to separate your daily habits into time bands that you can tick off easily. There are also additional videos, challenges and mindset hacks to help ingrain these habits into your daily life. It's colorful, musical and there's an element of community and competition with the app where you can converse with and challenge others.

Hiring a Coach

Checking in with a professional coach in the area of expertise of your goal is something I highly recommend.

Whether they be a fitness coach, nutritionist, business coach or sporting coach, there are so many dedicated professionals out there who help people achieve their goals and ambitions.

You might check in with a fitness professional with weekly weigh-in, measurements and progress pictures.

You might check in with a nutritionist with a weekly food diary.

You might check in with a business coach every week reporting back on the actions you have taken to grow and market your business.

Monitoring your progress will keep you motivated and maintain your goal-getting momentum but the additional beauty of hiring a coach is you benefit from their failure. A good coach has walked the path that you want to travel, or they have coached others to do the same with success. So always make sure you read testimonials and get proof of results.

With a good coach, they will teach you strategies for success and guide you on the right path. You do not have to experience the same pitfalls and as many inevitable bumps in the road that they did when you get professional help. When you invest in good quality coaching you are often pressing fast forward on your knowledge, goals and success.

Step 9

Rest, Relax and Reward

"Take a rest. A field that has rested gives a beautiful crop."
- Ovid

We have already touched on the need for sleep and rewards along the way to achieving our goals, but in this chapter, I want to dive into the importance of rest.

Firstly, when you start out on a path to success it can be difficult to gain the momentum needed to see your goals through to fruition. For example, if you're working towards a goal that is a year, five years or 'someday' away then it can be very easy to be derailed when a goal is so far out of reach, and you have a lot of work to put in to get there.

Rewarding yourself along the way for achieving milestones helps break up the goal into manageable pieces. These smaller goals are the necessary steps towards the large goals, and why shouldn't you reward yourself for your hard work, dedication and self-discipline?

Rewards have been ingrained in corporate business through targets, bonuses and promotion structures. It is why businesses thrive and remain profitable, otherwise what is the motivation?

It's the reason why it is important to introduce rewards for your own 'business' whether that is actually the business you have set up and are striving to grow, or the *business of you*. By that I mean, your own body, health, mindset and personal goals.

Rest

You've worked all week. You've not just burned the candle at both ends – you've blow torched it and there is nothing left in the tank. It's time to rest!

It can't all be push push push as we learned in the *Sprint vs Slow* chapter. We can't always have the 'on' switch on. We don't work like that.

It's really easy to ride the crest of a productivity wave and not factor in any rest.

What steps could you take to make sure it is incorporated into your weekly routine?

Digital Detox

A digital detox is a great way to give the old brain cells a rest. Detoxing from your devices one night a month (as an absolute minimum) is super valuable, especially if you live with other people or you have a family.

Could you try and incorporate a device free evening once a week to focus on true human connection? No TV, no iPads, no mobile phones or laptops. Get this in one night per week as a minimum and I promise you, there will be absolute creative gems that come to you in this time when your mind is not preoccupied and distracted by technology.

Sleep

There is a lot of focus on self-care in the media these days and the concept of a 'duvet day' where you assign one full day to the warmth of your duvet often feels like the holy grail of self-care practices. Some employers have the allowance of a number of duvet days in employee contracts. This is where, with no prior notice, you are allowed to call your employer and say that you are taking a duvet day as part of your pre-agreed paid or unpaid leave. In theory this can feel like a wonderful idea. Instead of employees calling in sick for ailments that might not truly prevent them from working, for example a hangover or feeling low, you can use a duvet day to rest with no need for self-certification of illness or a doctor's note.

Not every person will be able to just chuck the towel in and schedule in a duvet day. In some organisations it doesn't work at all due to the nature of workflow processes and many of us have commitments, careers and children to take care of. While it sounds like an ideal on paper, in reality it's not always that easy. However, if you have been feeling the pinch of exhaustion or your stress levels are high and your immune system feels run down, you could try and fit in a few early nights to help you refresh and recharge.

I challenge you reading this to try and go to bed one hour earlier every night for a week and notice how it makes you feel. Getting enough rest is associated with healthier body weight, greater motivation and smarter food choices. Sleep helps the brain to function much more efficiently, promotes learning, reduces stress, helps with problem solving and attention.

One way you can help yourself get to bed earlier each night is to set a bedtime alarm. Set it an hour before you want to go to sleep, have it go off and that be your signal to start your wind down. If you have a TV in your bedroom, unplug it at the wall for a week so the temptation to watch it is removed and notice if this helps you get to sleep earlier. Removing phones and tablets from your bedroom also helps and removes the temptation to scroll.

Revenge Bedtime Procrastination

I find it funny speaking about this topic as it is always the one we seem to find the hardest. In his book *Why We Sleep*, Matthew Walker reminds us that human beings are the only species that deliberately deprive themselves of sleep for no apparent gain.

There is a concept of 'revenge bedtime procrastination' that you might not have heard of before but I bet the majority of us do on a regular basis. Revenge bedtime procrastination is the act of purposely staying up late in order to steal back time. This may be due to a long and stressful day at work, engaging in activities forced upon you by others (a day at the in-law's house for example!), or parenting young children. Many people working long hours or parents who have battled their toddlers at bedtime will relate to this. When you feel like you have no social life or downtime, we try and reclaim our time through revenge bedtime procrastination. If you have worked from 9am to 9pm the best thing you could do for yourself is get a nutritious meal and then wind down for bedtime. But many of us feel so out of control with our schedules that we don't do this. Instead, we refuse to sleep early in order to regain some sense of freedom or control over our time into the late night hours.

Lack of Sleep and Heart Problems

Did you know? Every cell in the human body has an internal time mechanism according to Martin Young, Ph.D. in the University of Alabama at Birmingham Division of Cardiovascular Disease.

Martin Young has written many articles on the phenomenon of Daylight Savings and the clocks going forward an hour. The loss of an hour's sleep leads to an increased risk of heart attacks for people with a history of heart disease. When the clocks go forward by one hour in March, there is a 10-24 per cent increase in the risk of having a heart attack the following Monday!

This is due to the circadian clock – the body's internal time rhythms which occur over a 24 hour period. The internal circadian clock is responsible for driving rhythms in biological processes, responding to changes in light and dark in an organism's environment. When we disturb these natural rhythms with late nights, shorter mornings or something as simple as the clocks going forwards, our internal clocks don't have enough time to prepare our internal organs.

Scary stuff! So, it really is beneficial to get that extra hour of sleep in your rest tank, if you can. If you can make it your routine – even better!

Reward

Equally as important when striving towards your goals is the need for reward for completion, or rewards along the way.

I recently wanted to celebrate a year of sobriety and to mark the date looked at some beautiful engraved jewellery. I found it very difficult to commit to spending money on myself and almost didn't purchase it. If I had been buying this jewellery for a loved one or friend I would not have had any problem investing in it. Many of us struggle to spend on ourselves but honouring a goal achieved with some kind of symbolic gesture (even if it is something that doesn't cost money) is important to maintain your goal-getting motivation. Rewarding at milestones along the way makes the journey much more meaningful and enjoyable.

You might then be wondering how you can reward yourself along the way for milestones and mini goals that you achieve.

If your goal is a body composition goal and the reason you're reading this book to instill self- discipline when it comes to food and training, DON'T pick a food reward for hitting milestones. Pigging out on pizza or doughnuts is not getting you closer to your 'someday' goal and the short- term fix of sugar and comfort food is not beneficial to your long-term results.

If your goal is to hit a savings milestone, don't then reward yourself with something that will eat too much into said savings. You want to make this goal-getting journey as smooth and easy as possible.

Here's our guide to ways to reward yourself for your tenacity, self-discipline and goal-getting efforts:

1. Book a music concert for your favorite band
2. Learn a new skill and sign up for a class for something you have always wanted to learn
3. Have a proper duvet day off - stay in bed
4. Plan a mini holiday or short break with someone you love
5. Go for a night out with your friends
6. Organise a spa day
7. Get tickets to your favourite live sport
8. Throw a big party
9. See a movie in the middle of the day when the cinema is quiet
10. Get outside in nature; a walk, a bike ride, a picnic
11. Call or spend the day with a family member or friend who inspires you
12. Dance and sing (this does wonders for the soul!)
13. Enjoy a long hot bubble bath
14. Crack open a bottle of Champagne
15. Indulge in your favourite book
16. Host a board game night for you and your friends - no phones allowed!
17. Book the services of a personal shopper and buy clothes that suit your shape
18. Organise a photoshoot
19. Write a letter to a friend or family member you haven't connected with for a while

20. Book a session with a personal trainer
21. Arrange a beauty treatment
22. Book a nutrition assessment by a professional and get some meal plans drawn up
23. Test drive your dream car
24. Set yourself a challenge and book onto something like a running race, swim event, bike challenge or event like Tough Mudder
25. Begin a 'rewards saving' challenge where you reward yourself with money for every time you reach a certain goal.

There are so many different ways you can reward yourself along the way.

My personal favourite is the duvet day. I work so hard for such long periods, I love blocking out a day in my diary to do nothing. It works wonders for my creativity and energy levels and I truly feel like I've earned it when it happens.

Step 10

Failure v Success

"Our greatest glory is not in never failing, but in rising every time we fail."
- Confucius.

Thomas Edison, the inventor of the light bulb, tried over 1000 times to get a successful prototype of his invention that would go on to change all of our lives. A reporter later asked him "How did it feel to fail 1000 times?" to which he famously replied "I didn't fail 1000 times. The light bulb was an invention with 1000 steps."

Unlike Mr Edison, so many of us are petrified of failure and never even get started on our wildest dreams and goals for the fear that we won't reach them.

But how will you know unless you try?

We see it time and time again, so many people settle for mediocrity when there is no need to. If we could reach for our goals and not be held back by what scares us, how exciting would that prospect be?

I recently experienced an incredible two-day seminar by UK neuroscience and behaviour specialist Dax Moy. Dax is responsible for the deep transformation of his clients. He doesn't just change the way they look, but focuses on the physical, emotional and mental transformation of people thanks to his neuroscience methods which he blends with his fitness and nutrition training.

One thing stood out at that seminar, and it was these two phrases:

"Tolerate nothing."

"Desire everything or require nothing."

You should not have to tolerate situations in your life that bring about misery, clip your wings or stop you from achieving your potential. Whatever area of life it may be.

What are you tolerating? What are you putting up with that you don't need to? I'm not saying you should divorce your spouse or never speak to your sibling again, but what are you tolerating in your life that you could change? Where are you tolerating your excuses? Where are you blocking yourself and standing in your way?

You should desire to have it all. You CAN have it all. Put in the work, be strategic, be focused. Work on your steps to your goal with consistency, and you WILL get there. Even the smallest steps add up to monumental achievements when repeated consistently over time.

That is the magic secret of self-discipline or the compound effect of consistent action at the most basic and tiny level. My son and I were talking about him learning coding at school. "I would love to learn to code" I said to him. "Why don't you learn?" he replied. This got me thinking. I'd also had a conversation that day about small daily actions and we'd used learning a language as an example. If we learned one word a day in another language for a year, we'd know 365 words. Coding is like another language and if I learned one piece of code every day, I'd know 365 different coding commands in a year. You can use this rationale and thinking for anything. If you want to get better at absolutely anything in your life, start with one small action and repeat it consistently.

If you really think about it, the same effect happens the opposite way. If I were to make the decision to smoke a packet of cigarettes each day, drink a bottle of wine each night, get 4 hours of sleep per night then these actions would add up to some negative outcomes. I really believe that in creating new positive habits, we also get to undo and unpick some of the negative ones and reverse those decisions each day too. That's why I think I found giving up alcohol OK. It was a daily decision to not drink and over time it got easier to continue to say no to alcohol. The compound effect of the positive benefits on my heart health, skin, strength, finances and sleep helped me remain consistent with this one daily decision that went on to impact my life in such a positive way.

You Never Fail. You Always Learn

"Failure is not an option," NASA flight controller Jerry C. Bostick reportedly stated during the mission to bring the damaged Apollo 13 back to Earth. That phrase has been etched into the collective memory ever since.

If you don't try, you won't know. You see, failure is life's greatest teacher. When you deem yourself to have 'failed' what can this perceived 'failure' actually teach you? What lessons can you learn?

Failure is one of the most powerful tools in reaching great success. Consider the greatest thinkers of our time; Einstein, Darwin, Freud, business mavericks and sporting legends all had the bravery to fly above the radar, go against the grain, make the waves, attract the attention and carve a path to success. Did they fail along the way? Of course!

Many modern-day employers embrace failure. Blue-chip companies are known to seek out those who have experienced failure alongside success. Those employees who have been on both sides of the failure and success coin bring valuable and essential experience along to the party. They can demonstrate resilience, responsibility, perseverance, and the wounds to show they have survived the business battle and lived to tell the tale.

To be competitive, to meet targets, to stay ahead of the competition, you have to stick your neck out on the line every single day. This is the same for your non-business, more personal goals you're on the way to achieving. You have to push hard, think big and block out the fear of failure.

Perceived failure, while often painful at the time, can result in our greatest personal growth. When we consider our failures of the past, once we are out of the possible pain of those failures, we can retrospectively look back and see the gifts in those things that went wrong.

It's a little superficial, but here goes. My 60lb weight gain after my breakdown was painful at times, and I definitely deemed it as a failure at some points. The gift of failing and piling on weight is that I have learned to love and accept my body. I realised I'd made drastic changes, and I had to work with what I had. I wasn't going to shed the weight overnight and instead of starving myself or embarking on a gruelling exercise plan, I was supported through a period of self-love and learned to accept who I am right now in any given moment. I have realised that I am the type of person that needs to take it one day and one action at a time when it comes to goals, and I've been able to see the patterns of past attempts and where I went wrong. As a result, I learn, take the lessons and grow.

Recently I worked for a client who had suffered a business collapse a few years ago. We spoke at length about his former business, and he was still very much hurt from the pain of losing his livelihood, laying people off and selling assets like his car. Even though he recalled this episode of his life with sadness, he said it was the best lesson he learned in his entrepreneurial journey. His whole company ran on a specific piece of government policy that was never guaranteed to be around forever. The new government was elected, the policy abolished and the business lasted three months before it folded. Now he strives to have different sources of income within his company and never entirely rely on one revenue stream.

Another contact of mine was declared bankrupt in his early twenties. Just through being young, getting too much credit and then not having the means to live and pay off his loans, he didn't admit it to anyone until it was too late and bankruptcy was the only option. Now, this might be perceived as a failure, but you talk to him honestly about it, and he will tell you it is the best thing that ever happened in his life. Two decades later, his attitude to money took on a new life after bankruptcy, and he works to help others never experience this and save for the future.

Reframe Your Failures

Reframing your failures is a powerful exercise. This can help you let go of the baggage of perceived failures and understand the gifts in not achieving past goals.

Think about three goals you've 'failed' at in your life.

Write down all the gifts that this failure brought you. You could do this as a diary entry and set a timer to write about it, or here are some helpful journal prompts that might be beneficial:

What did you learn by not achieving this goal?

What did failing at this goal mean for you?

What was the lesson that this failure made you realise?

Is that goal still important to you?

What could you do (or what did you do) differently in the future to go on to achieve that goal?

Transformation is about growth and you can't grow without failure because nothing will ever go right the first time and nothing will ever be perfect. Being able to draw a line under the challenges and the hard times and take the lessons to pivot, adapt and grow is one of the greatest traits in people and one that will help you reach your intended goal destination.

Conclusion

How is it possible to get two people training for a marathon where one designs a training plan and prepares in advance while the other procrastinates on action and wings it on the day?

Or two people want to get out of debt. One adjusts their budget and saves over time, the other struggles to maintain the action steps needed to keep an eye on their money and separate cash out for savings.

Or how about two people both trying to lose weight, at a restaurant perusing the menu and one orders the salad while the other says "I wish I had your willpower".

Willpower doesn't exist. It is a phenomenon that is fictitious. Self-discipline is not something that you are born with; it is something that is *learned*.

You can learn it too. I promise.

Delayed Gratification

In this fast-paced, easy financed and aspirational digital world we live in, we don't really possess a lot of patience. When our grandparents were young, if they wanted something, like an extravagant purchase, they would have to save and save until they could afford it.

When our grandparents were in their youth clothes were hand made, food was grown in the garden and meals were cooked from scratch. They didn't have Uber Eats to satisfy their hunger every weekend!

I went to school in the 90s, and if I wanted to research a certain topic, I would have to go to the library and read book after book, taking pages of notes. These days the answers are at a click of a button thanks to the internet.

Our international culture of credit, our fast food and having access to all the answers to all our questions means we have lost the art of patience.

In turn, we have lost the art of self-discipline and delaying gratification for the greater good.

There is a very well documented test and study involving children and marshmallows, demonstrating how delayed gratification plays out to a young child. The study's essence is a child is seated at a table, and a single marshmallow is placed on a plate in front of them. The adult leading the study sits them down, shows the marshmallow and explains that they can choose to either eat the marshmallow now, or wait until they come back, not eat it, and they will get research marshmallows to eat.

If you research this test, it has been repeated many times throughout many countries and is always fascinating and entertaining to watch these small 4 or 5-year-old children practise self-discipline and self-restraint in order to wait it out and get the extra marshmallow.

Some kids just ate the marshmallow straight away. Other kids were quite ingenious and got around the rules and hardship of waiting it out by sniffing the marshmallows, licking them, nibbling one side and then trying to hide the bite marks. Some kids noticeably demonstrated restraint and self-discipline by actively trying to distract themselves from the marshmallow by looking around, swinging their legs or shutting their eyes. For those children who showed self-discipline and delayed gratification, they were rewarded with an additional marshmallow.

This original study was conducted in the 1960s but a 1972 follow-up study by Walter Mischel from Stanford University yielded the most surprising results. Mischel followed up with many of the children who had taken part in the original study. From the original marshmallow test results, Mischel was able to see that of the children who waited it out, therefore delaying gratification to get their second marshmallow, a high percentage had higher exam results, lower levels of substance abuse, lower incidence of obesity, were better equipped to deal with stress and generally reported to have better social skills by their parents.

The children from the original study, the ones who had not been able to resist the temptation of the marshmallows, achieved lower grades, reported more substance abuse and were more likely to be obese in comparison to their self-disciplined peers.

Right now, in this present moment, you might feel that you're not that great at delaying gratification. I know I wasn't. I'd be the kid scoffing the marshmallow within seconds! Yet the methods and strategies outlined in this book have been a life-saver for me in my own quest and that of others I have taught to help them feel healthier, happier and more successful.

My clients and community have taken inspiration from the methods outlined in this book and have reported feeling more organised, focused, less stressed and have achieved many goals.

Research suggests that you can certainly improve your self-discipline and ability to delay gratification by adopting a few simple steps. I hope you are able to take something away from this book and adopt even just a couple of steps to help you improve your self-discipline.

Truth Bomb Alert!!!

I really struggle with self-discipline. So do many people I have helped to increase their willpower through the repetition of discipline and building habits.

It doesn't come naturally to a lot of people. Many people have to force it. I know I'm not the only one! Self-discipline is something that many people do have to force out of their system. I know it takes me a considerable amount of effort to get out of the starting blocks, but once I do, I'm away and sprinting to the goal-getting finish.

I have spent so much time and finances on learning how to have more self-discipline in my life, to then ingrain positive habits and live a life that feels like I'm in control.

I've loved passing on what I have learned to my readers, clients, friends and family. I've helped people to not *just* change, but truly transform and not *just* achieve their goals, but smash them out of the water quicker, easier and with more enjoyment.

Focusing on self-discipline for the book and teaching many of these points to others had a positive and knock-on effect in many other areas of my life. Even though my natural tendency is to want to rebel against rigid discipline, I know that staying on top of those mundane tasks, having a solid morning routine and focusing on daily decisions has changed me and made life easier.

I really feel like writing this book was a gift to me and it has been my stepping stone to share the gifts of discipline with others. I no longer feel like I "should have a PhD in Procrastination" as I used to joke about a lot. I learned about self-discipline by forcing myself into action until my brain realised that this way of living made life happier, easier and a lot less stressed.

For me, this self-discipline journey was about developing self-trust. I hadn't realised how much I was programmed to feel like I'd fail anyway when aiming for goals. With every small act of discipline, I started to build self-trust, and once that was cemented in my mindset, my whole belief system changed. I love now going through this same process with my 1:1 and group mentoring clients. I love speaking about this at events and in groups. It is so moving to watch the light bulbs go off for people when they realise that discipline can be reframed into beautiful and powerful promises to yourself, that you keep. I want people to develop discipline for a lifetime, not just for a 16-week transformation challenge. I want to help people realise that there are ebbs and flows of life and you will never ever be 'on it' 100% all the time. I want people to embrace their flaws and failures, learn all about themselves, play to their energy type and cut themselves some slack.

I often say that the gift is actually in messing up.

When you mess up, and when you analyse that messing up, you realise what went wrong. The important part is to not dwell on that perceived 'failure' but put on your big grown-up pants, take responsibility, dust yourself off and think "What would I do differently next time?"

That's the power of these methods for achieving self-discipline in 10 steps. While you focus on your one thing and achieve your big goals with small daily action steps, you'll find you naturally gravitate to unconsciously improving other areas of your life.

After all, another of my favourite phrases always triggers me in good ways and bad:

"How you do *one* thing is how you do *every*thing."

When you start doing one thing in a way that benefits your life, it naturally starts to leak into other areas too. It's a positive upward trajectory of building new habits that make life easier.

I look forward to everything falling into place for you, overcoming procrastination and achieving your own goals.

Remember, you make your own luck. Go get em!

Gemma Ray

A Gift for Every Reader to Help You Take Action

Bonus #1 - Goal Setting Masterclass and Companion Workbook
Enjoy the Goal Setting Masterclass and accompanying workbook that will really help you to understand what you want to achieve, why you want to achieve it and then be able to confidently outline the action steps you can take to achieve your goals.

Bonus #2 – 60 Minute Procrastination Busting Guided Focus Audio
Need to focus? Get my 60-minute procrastination busting guided focus audio. This follows the Pomodoro method and will help keep you on track when trying to concentrate.

Simply visit **www.gemmaray.com/selfdiscipline** to get instant access to the masterclass, workbook and guided productivity audio.

For further reading, publications and additional resources, please visit **www.gemmaray.com**

Final Note – Did you enjoy the book? If so, can you help?

As a self-published author duo, my accountability buddy Ben and I had to learn everything about self-publishing from scratch. This book would not be in your hands now had we not developed a plan to learn all we could about Amazon, Audible, self-publishing, formatting, technical specs, Kindle coding, cover designs etc. It's been a mammoth task, but it has made us better people.

We don't have the powerhouse of a publishing company and a team of experts to launch and market our book for us. We rely on word of mouth recommendation and reviews on platforms such as Amazon, Audible and Goodreads. We do all the work ourselves in between our jobs and lives and have no additional staff. It's just us!

If you have enjoyed the book, we would appreciate you sparing a minute to leave us a positive review. Every independent review helps us spread the message we are trying to share about self-discipline and how it has truly helped us improve our lives.

You can leave a review here: **mybook.to/selfdiscipline** or at **www.goodreads.com**

Thank you. We hope to connect with you in the Facebook group or work with you in one of our upcoming Mastermind groups.

STOP PROCRASTINATING START LIVING

Beat Procrastination and Boost Productivity for Self Care and Success

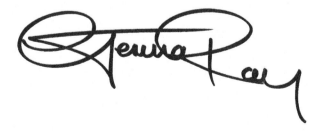

Copyright © 2020 Gemma Ray

All rights reserved. This book or any portion thereof may not be reproduced or used in any manner whatsoever without the express written permission of the publisher except for the use of brief quotations in a book review.

Other books by Gemma Ray

2020 - Stop Procrastinating and Start Living: Beat Procrastination and Boost Productivity for Self Care and Success

www.gemmaray.com

For my friend Michelle, who squeezed every precious moment out of life every day.

Praise for *Stop Procrastinating and Start Living*

"Brilliant book. Well written. Useful tips, with practical examples of how you can overcome procrastination not only in your work life, but in changes you want to make in your personal life too. I read it over 3 days and will definitely be going back to it next time I find myself procrastinating."

–Jacky Hodges

"Gemma has put together a tool box jam packed with tips and advice on how to make real sustainable lifestyle changes that can be easily adapted to anyone's circumstances. Since being a beta reader for Stop Procrastinating Start Living my life has completely changed. I've stopped drinking and stuck to a diet plan easily losing 13lbs in a few weeks. I can't believe it!"

–Hayley Goulding

"In this follow-up to her excellent debut 'Self Discipline', Gemma has distilled her extensive background research and combined it with tried and tested tips, creating an accessible and highly practical guide. Written in her fun and approachable style, there is something in here for everyone who is looking to overcome procrastination in any area of their life and boost their well-being."

–Karen Dequatre Cheeseman

"I'm known to my friends as the one who gets stuff done but the secret is that I wake up feeling stuck regularly - in this book, Gemma provides the antidote. Think of it as the ultimate remedy for every possible procrastinating scenario. Bold claim, I know, but seriously no matter what goal you're working towards right now, Gemma has the tools and advice to help you make that happen

and she's sharing them all in this book in her down-to-earth, lovely Gemma way."
—Daire Paddy, Brain & Business Coach

"Wow, I absolutely loved it! Very motivational. I liked the mixture of scientific evidence plus personal experience. I loved the practical exercises."
—Michelle Leathley

"This book seems like it was written for me. My biggest takeaway is accepting that I'm not just lazy, I'm not the only person behaving this way and that I'm perfectly ok. Can I be better? Yes and thanks to habit stacking, I am already better than I was. Read it. Pick something. Do it. It's that simple."
—Geraldine Morey

Gifts from Me to You

As a thank you for downloading this book I would like to give you a free gift that I know will complement and strengthen the strategies outlined in this book.

Free Goal Setting Masterclass

This powerful session will help you get clear on your goals. When you know what you are aiming for and the meaningful reasons why, it gives you clarity.

Free Goal Setting Masterclass Workbook

It's easy to watch a masterclass but harder to implement the strategies, so follow the plan and the workbook.

Get your free gifts at: **www.gemmaray.com/bonus**.

Prologue

Procrastination is like the friend your parents always disapproved of you hanging out with. You loved your endless, reckless time together but you also knew they acted like a really bad influence. There are times when you and your friend 'Procrastination' don't see each other for a while as you get super focused on other things. Sometimes seeing each other is a real treat after a period of long, hard work. The moments you're together, you're carefree and time seems to stand still. On some occasions you hang out a bit too much. You even skip work to get together and procrastination has the power to get you into trouble or neglect really important areas of your life. Procrastination isn't a fan of being healthy, or working hard or studying. It's like you just "Got in with the wrong crowd" as your friend procrastination gradually drags you down.

You don't want to get rid of procrastination out of your life entirely. You know that's not possible. The two of you have been buddies for a long time and when your relationship is in a healthy place, it can be really good for you to hang out. Procrastination can help you wind down, take a break, relax and it loves to help you overthink lots of weird and wonderful things. When your relationship turns toxic and procrastination has a control over you that threatens your health, your job, your studies and your relationships - that's the time to take some action.

Taking action is difficult when procrastination has become an almost conjoined twin of yours. You intertwine so easily, which is the exact reason I urge you to sit with your friend procrastination a little while and enjoy this book in the company of one another. Use your time together to read through each chapter and test out the many different theories, strategies and suggestions. You'll probably find you'll separate for a while as you work through the chapters in the book and test out the science-based strategies steeped in psychology and neuroscience. Some strategies will appeal to you. They'll resonate with your lifestyle, the way you work, your studies, your sporting ambitions or your health goals. They'll wake you up to the reality that your encounters with procrastination are taking you away from your dreams and all you are capable of. Some of the exercises will help you pull away gently from the grasp of procrastination so you can stress less, reduce your overwhelm and stop feeling anxious. This book will help guide you into the embrace of focus, productivity, achievement, pride, wealth, happiness and purpose.

Introduction

Is Self Discipline the Highest Form of Self Care?

Overcoming procrastination takes practice and discipline. You must first practice different coping methods when procrastination strikes to help you become more focused and productive. Practicing these methods consistently and finding the strategies that work for you will become a habit, making procrastination easier to manage over time. Being in a position to put these methods into practice requires discipline. If you want to achieve a sporting goal, you require an initial burst of self-discipline to train and the continued desire to practice which means you take action. If you want to write a book, you require the initial discipline to sit down and write and the continued practice of consistent research and writing. If you want to make 100 sales this month you require the initial discipline to outline your sales pitch and target customers and the continued practice of making yourself and your sales message visible to your target leads and selling to them. Repeated action yields goal success.

I was recently asked to deliver a keynote speech on my own journey with self discipline. I was a little nervous speaking to this particular audience about self discipline as the attendees of the event were very spiritual in their approach. In their world (and mine too) we believe in being guided by intuition, not having to force aspects of our lives and believing that the Universe has our backs. I like to think this way. I am not a religious person but I admire those who are as they have something to believe in to help them believe in themselves. I draw a similar line of thought by my own views on belief that there is something greater out there for me that has my best interests at heart. Yet practicing discipline, working hard and also believing in pushing myself in the 'hustle and grind' right now to have a freer life later is also a strong personal belief. I needed a way to marry the two schools of thought that would appeal to this audience and this was it;

"Is self discipline the highest form of self care?"

This was the big takeaway question I asked the audience.

Self love has been a big theme in recent years across social media. In the shadows of the #MeToo movement, women are rising up against unrealistic body expectations and embracing a whole body positivity message that we should love and accept ourselves as we are. As someone who had put on a lot of weight and someone who has worked for fitness and nutrition professionals for the past seven years, I really wanted to be a part of this movement. I wanted to love my body and embrace it for all it is. I tried so hard staring in the mirror, wobbling my jiggly bits and practicing gratitude for the body that had birthed my son and the body I'd abused with food and alcohol for far too long. The body I had struggled to allow enough time to sleep and adequately recover from everyday stresses and strains. I actively worked on my own self love and self worth issues, noticing my reaction to my reflection in the mirror, reminding myself "I am enough" and doing a lot of work with coaches on increasing my inner confidence.

I felt better. There's no doubt about it. I was looking at my reflection with more love and acceptance and it felt like a nice place to be. Inside my own head was a happier and more fulfilled place than it had been in a long time. But something still wasn't right. Something was still off when I tried so hard to practice self love and self acceptance. I finally figured it out. It was all very well embracing my curves and extra weight, dressing for my actual shape rather than attempting to squeeze into ill-fitting clothing and feeling sad at my reflection, but I wasn't fully loving myself for one really important reason. I wasn't doing enough. I had the phrase "I am enough" written on the mirrors in my home and I even looked into getting it tattooed on my wrist. It was a really powerful statement that instantly made me feel good, but just as quick as those feelings of acceptance and self love rushed through my veins, the feeling of fakeness and being false presented in the way I looked back at myself. It was really hard to say "I am enough" to myself in the mirror when the cold hard facts were that I wasn't actually doing enough to make me feel like that statement was true. I was too wrapped up trying to fit into a body positivity movement that told me I was fine as I am. Eat all the food. Don't exercise. Just dance in your pants on social media and everyone will comment how 'brave' and 'inspiring' you are. It just felt wrong. If I were a very slim woman with an athletic or slender figure, dancing in my underwear and plastering it on social media would brand me an attention seeker. Just because I'm larger doesn't mean I'm brave. I felt like the use of this word actually meant "It's not the norm or attractive for someone with your curvy non-magazine perfect body shape to dance around in your underwear leaving yourself to everyone's judgement - so you are brave." It felt like a cop out. Carrying on the way I was; binge eating, not exercising, prioritising work over everything else wasn't making me feel good on the inside and I felt it reflected on how I looked on the outside. So I fell out with the body positivity movement and its permission to procrastinate on exercise and good nutrition. I decided I needed to go back to the drawing board and figure out what self care and self love looked like for me.

For some people self care is bubble baths, massages, a guilt free Netflix binge, a night out with the girls, an early night, meditation or a journaling session. I love all of those things and if I were to draw up a first aid kit of self care for myself, they would probably all feature in there. However, these methods were often used as ways to procrastinate on tasks and certain actions that my future self would thank me for. It all seemed OK and excusable though. We all need self care and self love, right? But when is too much self care and not enough genuine self love an excuse and another form of procrastination?

In November 2019 I decided to embark on a crazy self discipline challenge. My first book was written all about self discipline but I felt like a fraud. I was disciplined in so many areas of my life - particularly around my work but I wasn't disciplined in any area of my life that focused on my health and well-being, so I decided to take drastic action. Called #75Hard[1] and developed by Andy Frisella, the founder of 1st Phorm supplement company, this self discipline challenge was dubbed "The way to win the tactical war on yourself". The challenge was 75 days in duration and involved me working out twice a day with one session outdoors no matter the weather, drinking a gallon of water, reading self development books and picking a diet and sticking to it. If you fail on any of the daily tasks which also included a daily progress picture, you went back to the beginning and started again. I'd seen other friends attempt this and a search of the #75Hard hashtag on social media showed me many happy people who had completed the 10 week process and reported how much it had helped them mentally. So I went for it. I walked everywhere I could, averaging around 6 miles a day. I drank my water and read my books. I didn't drink a drop of alcohol and water became my best friend. I was adding in around two hours worth of extra stuff a day but feeling like I had more time. I was focused, I had a purpose and I was doing it! By the third week of the challenge something really changed inside of me. I looked in the mirror (where 'I am enough' was still written in fancy cursive chalk pen) and I believed the girl who looked back at me for the first time in years. I was enough. Truly. I believed it for the first time and felt emotional. I was starting to believe in myself. Why was that? Why was doing this ridiculous challenge shifting something so deep rooted inside me? I realised that I had tried and failed many many times over the last four years to keep my promises to myself. They might have been really small things like "I'll get to the gym three times this week" or "I'll track my calories tomorrow" or "I'll stop eating crisps at lunch" but I'd made countless of these promises and hardly kept any of them. What happens when you don't keep your promises to yourself? You lose trust in yourself. What happens when you lose trust in yourself? You lose belief in yourself.

All of this cycle of failure was keeping me stuck and my self worth was pretty low. It had been like this for a long time by this point and it's no surprise my procrastination powers had also dramatically increased. When you feel crap about yourself and you feel like you're going to fail anyway, getting motivated to even start is a hard slog. I was at the mercy of procrastination every single day and it was causing me untold stress and overwhelm. As soon as I started to adopt the #75Hard actions into my daily routine, I started to keep my promises to myself and was learning the art of keeping procrastination at bay. Getting out first thing and walking in the crisp winter air woke up my body and my mind so that returning to work from my home office became easier. I got into my work routine quicker and made great progress on my tasks. I meal-prepped in advance, sticking to the diet I set for myself which saved time and stress and gave me more mental energy to focus on other more important stuff. Reading before bed (which was part of the challenge) helped me stay off social media and helped me sleep quicker. Being able to fit in the workouts required forward planning so I became a master at time management and was getting a lot of my work done a lot quicker, knowing I had to be out the door to walk to school and pick up my son in time. Even just getting outside in the fresh air helped my mental health. In the 10 weeks I adopted #75Hard routines, I had no anxiety or depression. I felt level headed and happy.

It was a lot to fit into my life and I wouldn't recommend it to everyone. There were plenty of times I was walking in the pitch black in freezing temperatures with sleet and hailstones stinging my face wondering what the hell I was doing. I didn't drink over Christmas and I even arrived at a New Year party an hour late as I walked there in my party outfit - just to get my workout in! My family thought I was crazy but I needed something drastic to get me out of the procrastination hole I'd been hiding in. During my 75 days of the challenge I also put the final touches to this very book you are reading now. I tripled my income on my first book and doubled my income in my day-to-day client work. I lost 19lbs in the process (although

I didn't focus on this too much - it was a positive side effect) and I dramatically reduced my bloated waistline. I slept more. I went on social media less and I really kicked my procrastination tendencies to the curb. I felt like I'd found the magic pill for productivity but at the same time knew it wasn't something I could continue for the long term. My husband was worried about me heading out walking in the dark every night and it did take me away from my mum duties. My son also hated walking home from school in the rain and moaned that he hadn't signed up to the challenge so why was I making him do it too? When my 75 days were up, I had considered doing it all over again but decided that was it for me, I was done. I had proved to myself I was capable and could fit in a lot more than I realised - especially when I was no longer procrastinating! I also proved I could keep my promises to myself.

The biggest takeaway of this whole process for me was that self care and self love looks different for me. I can do bubble baths and yoga a bit too easily and actually use them as an excuse to not take action. "Oh I am tired, I will have this bath because I need to do my self care routine" is an unhelpful reason for self care if you have a pile of work that needs to be finished, you're putting it off until tomorrow, and it's going to just add to your future mental stress. I realised that looking in the mirror and having true body positivity comes when you respect and honour your body enough with consistent nurture through good food, fresh air and moving your body in a way that excites you and makes you happy. Being able to look at my body in the mirror with a genuine smile of self love and self appreciation only came when I started to take action. The feeling of pride replaced the feeling of self loathing and it felt very alien but also very moving.

The same happened with my mental health. Understanding that taking action today will help 'future me' was a revelation. I was too familiar with procrastinating on too many things, leaving actions until the last minute and then causing future me untold misery, stress, upset and worry. I'd suffered from anxiety and had panic attacks on occasions - all not helped by me putting things off until I was left in a position where I had no choice other than to take action and take it immediately. Learning to take the smallest of steps on certain projects, tasks and actions was pure relief. No longer was I using precious mental energy by just thinking about the actions I needed to take, I was taking small actions which actually stopped the thinking and worrying. I had things covered. I felt more in control. I didn't feel stressed and anxious.

The reality is that living this way with a regimented approach to discipline goes against who I am as a free-spirited person. It's boring and I hate feeling like I have to force myself out of a procrastination state in order to focus and get stuff done, but when I do get stuff done I realise how valuable my self-discipline has been in order to get me moving and motivated. I have a lot I want to achieve. If I want to stop with the discipline I must also accept that I won't be able to see what my true potential is and that's not an option for me. I am a high achiever and always have been, so to keep achieving high I need to do the things that work for me to get me into a state of focus, motivation and excitement for the tasks ahead. I have come to realise for me self-discipline is the highest form of self love. Doing the hard stuff today makes life for me in the future a lot easier. Which is why I have made it my mission to spread the word of self-discipline to the dreamers, thinkers, creatives and free spirits like myself. It is not something that comes naturally to me, but when I practice it, when I work on banishing procrastination and really seeing how productive I can be - that's when the magic happens. That's when I find my purpose.

As much as I resist it, I know it works. Using methods to increase productivity and being disciplined in my thoughts and actions has helped me save my marriage, be a better mum, build my dream home, realise my dreams of being an author, increase my income, improve my mental health, like what I see in the mirror, trust myself and believe in myself again. I am happier and healthier when I actively work on banishing procrastination and wrote this book because I want this for you too.

Change can happen in an instant and every one of us can make a decision to change. My friend Helen posted online today about making a split second decision to start a new health and fitness regime. She said "Change doesn't need to be complex. Change happens in an instant." It's been on my mind all day. She's spot on. Because that's what change actually is. It is a decision made in one single moment which is followed up with action. It isn't about achieving the end result, but rather being mentally resilient enough to make a decision that is a positive and helpful change - even if it feels difficult. You get to do that right now. You get to decide you want to make a change for the better and then use this book to explore ways that might help you change and shift you out of procrastination and into being productive.

A pre-warning to you, dear reader, and a heartfelt request

WARNING Many things you will read in this book will contradict one another. When you write about a topic which affects us all, you widen the potential audience. When you widen the potential audience, you really can't satisfy every single reader. Therefore, I'd really urge you to take from each chapter what appeals to you and ignore the tips that you know won't work for your own personal circumstances, lifestyle, personality type and goals. One recent negative review on my last book, Self Discipline, gave me a 1 star rating because "You can find all this stuff out on the internet." No shit Sherlock! You really can. In the same way you could buy all your own ingredients and cook at home instead of eating a meal prepared by a chef in a restaurant. Or you could read up on the best way to colour your hair instead of visiting a hairdresser. Or you could read about all the latest diets instead of joining a diet club or hiring a personal trainer.

Being a journalist and a writer is about using research from experts, books, audio and video channels, scientific studies and using your own experiences to pull together engaging content. This book is just that. A culmination of six months of deep research, four tireless and life changing years of self testing, coaching others in the methods and bringing it all together into an easy-to-read format. I don't do big complicated words and jargon littered literature. I do straight talking, honest and no nonsense advice that I hope will inspire you into action.

I'm also a woman. I felt it was important to point this out because I don't know of many famous female authors that talk about productivity and procrastination. In a recent list of 100 recommended books published in a discipline group I'm part of[2], I was really sad to see that not one was written by a woman. That doesn't mean that I have a soft approach and I'm not at the other popular productivity and discipline extreme of ex-military. What I am is a safe pair of hands for any man, woman or teenager looking to be guided to feel more fulfilled in their work, health, passions and lives through the productivity methods I've explored in the book.

How the book works

Step 1: Procrastinate by reading the book

Don't worry, the irony is not lost on me that this is a book about the very thing you need to stop doing to even read the book in the first place. If easier, commit to something small like reading 10 pages every day. You'll read it within the month.

Step 2: Forgive yourself

I want you to feel forgiveness for all the negativity that has been caused by procrastination so far in your life. We will delve into this more in the book but for now, take this sentence as your permission slip to draw a line under your procrastination so far, pause your pressing tasks and read this book.

Step 3: Read the WHOLE BOOK first

Eventually when you have read this whole book in its entirety, you will be able to come back to it time and time again, flick through the pages and land on something magical to immediately pull you out of your procrastination hole.

Before you get to that point though, read the whole book first. Procrastinate on it (I'm telling you again in case you missed me say it the first time). See it as an investment. Waste a bit of time on the tasks you should be doing by reading this book. Once you have read it, I guarantee something in it will have inspired you and the time and energy you'll get back coupled with the reduced stress levels will be worth it.

This book is going to make you think about YOU and your behaviours. It will get you to think about your habits, your actions and who you believe yourself to be. It will get you to assess and audit how you work and think to come up with a strategy that helps you THE NEXT TIME you find procrastination ruining your life.

So invest the time to read this book. Get thinking about the stuff that comes up in each chapter and how it relates to you. Create a plan that works for you completely before you toss this book in the downstairs bathroom for your guests to flick through.

Step 4: Flick through it whenever procrastination is being a bitch

When procrastination is being a complete little bitch and she's knocking at your door, this is when you need this book. When she's telling you to binge watch that latest series on Netflix, rearrange your cutlery drawer or mess around on Facebook for the next two hours (when really you need to get that report sent off before you get fired) then get this book, flick through to a random page and follow the anti-procrastination instructions.

I wanted to create a guide book that would help those of us living in this harsh real world to be supported to take responsibility. This is a mature and sensible guide for anyone putting any task off in their life. Take this book, flick through it and use the advice as a little sign, a little magic, a push on an imaginary procrastination panic button that will help you get off your ass, get going and feel great again.

Step 5: Take what you need, discard what you don't

We are all different. Some of us have corporate careers, others run their own businesses. Some are students, some are retired. Some are parents, some are too young to even think about a family. We all have different challenges and things pulling our attention in so many different directions. Not every chapter will resonate with you but I urge you to try as much as you can and enjoy experimenting while working out what works for you.

Step 6: Utilise the affirmations and journal prompts

In every chapter I have included affirmations and journal prompts for you. If these affirmations resonate with you, you may choose to repeat them to yourself, or write them somewhere prominent for you to see. I am a huge fan of journaling so have provided different journaling prompts for you to explore in your own journal writing sessions. Again, both of these tools have been provided as suggestions and are entirely optional. If you are using this book in times of trying to get out of procrastination immediately, I hope the affirmations and journal prompts will provide useful and help you change your mental state so you feel ready to take action. I truly believe the answers to every time we stall are within us and really encourage you to give the journaling a go.

Many of us say we are just "trying to find a balance" when it comes to our home lives, families, work lives and passions/hobbies. Some people are able to accept their own procrastinating tendencies and continue their lives as normal. For others, like me, it eats away at your self worth, self belief and self trust causing you untold stress and misery.

I can't lie to you and tell you I have this all figured out. I really don't. I am so proud of what I have achieved despite my internal monkey mind trying to sabotage my efforts. I struggle with procrastination every single day in some form and I'm so happy to say that every single day it also gets a little easier to manage. Even if 'easier' looks like forgiving myself, drawing a line under what has been and focusing on the future action I can take rather than dwelling on my past negative inaction.

That's what this book is all about. Moving on. Forgiving yourself. Learning about yourself and your own energy patterns, discovering your limiting beliefs, carving out your own productivity style and other factors that make you the unique human being that you are. Just remember that truly magnificent, intriguing and powerful brain of yours can make a decision to change in a split second. It is within your power to make that decision right now.

For more information on anti procrastination tools including journal prompts, planners and audio programmes please visit **www.gemmaray.com**.

Chapter 1

What is Procrastination Anyway?

What *is* procrastination anyway?

Breaking down the word procrastination, 'pro' means *forward, forth, in favour of* or *the future* and 'crastinus' means *tomorrow*. Or a modern day translation might be "I'll do it tomorrow."

It is an undesired delay, the act of putting off things that are really important in favour of less urgent tasks or to actively engage in more pleasurable activity over less pleasurable expectations, promises or tasks. It is knowing exactly what we want to achieve in the future, while taking no action in the present moment to actually make that future achievement a reality.

Solving the procrastination problem is developing the ability to forego immediate gratification for the sake of long term achievement. It is the art of becoming less impulsive and easily sidetracked. We can all be the person who chooses fun in the moment and what feels good right now over what is not as fun but will pay off in the future. It is an avoidance technique that is a natural part of human existence.

Procrastination is not something new. It has been written about throughout history with one of the earliest references to procrastination in the poem 'Work and Days' by Greek poet Hesiod[1] circa 800BC. In the verse, written with annoyance at his brother Perses, he writes:

"Do not put your work off till tomorrow and the day after; For a sluggish worker does not fill

his barn, nor one who puts off his work: Industry makes work go well, but a man who puts off work is always at hand-grips with ruin."

In The Canterbury Tales[2], Geoffrey Chaucer's 14th century writing observes Dame Prudence say to Melibee and his associates, *"...the goodness you may do this day, do it; and delay it not until tomorrow."* Ironic words from the greatest English poet of the Middle Ages who originally planned 100 Canterbury Tales but only published 24 before his death[3]. Still an incredible literary achievement that continues to inspire to this day.

The world's most famous painting - The Mona Lisa, by Leonardo Da Vinci, took 16 years to complete![4] We'll let old Leonardo off though. He may have procrastinated for a decade and a half on Mona Lisa's side smile but he also worked on sketching inventions way ahead of his era including a 15th century helicopter.

The modern day procrastinator is bombarded with distractions from all angles. Whether it be social media, phone calls, texts, emails, app notifications for all areas of life, it is difficult to keep focused in a world overflowing with information so easily at our fingertips. Over 20 years ago, when I studied for my high school exams, I had to make trips to the library and pore over books to find the answers to my questions. Now, since the age of only three years old, my son has been asking the technology in our home to give him the answers to all his questions. These answers arrive at lightning speed. Our hands have direct access to the answer to any question and our heads are completely full, overwhelmed and struggling to process the onslaught of information at our disposal.

When you go to our friend Google and ask *'What is procrastination?'* you see other questions in the same genre appear. One of the common accompanying suggestions is *'Is procrastination a mental disorder?'.*

I found myself mildly triggered seeing that question. We ALL procrastinate in some form or another. That doesn't mean we all have a mental disorder. Does it?

Surprisingly, procrastination can be linked to certain psychological disorders such as depression, irrational behaviour, low self esteem, anxiety and neurological disorders like ADHD[5]. Patients with neurological injury in the prefrontal cortex area of the brain or those with an imbalance in the frontal lobe can often be plagued by a myriad of different psychological, neurological and self esteem challenges with procrastination being a symptom of impaired impulse responses.

You might have had a brain injury, illness or trauma that has caused your neurological function to weaken. Your prefrontal cortex damage may have affected your ability to foresee future scenarios to process present choices.

The way we feel about ourselves and within ourselves can factor where we sit on the procrastination severity scale. Low self esteem, anxiety and depression can sometimes cause a feeling of hopelessness and helplessness with procrastination becoming a symptom. You might feel similar. You might have suffered from depression or continue to live with the black dog of depression and resonate with the symptoms of not having the "get up and go" to get things done. That is completely understandable and normal.

There are some people who suffer so badly from procrastination that it can affect all areas of their life. In the same way that you can't just tell a depressed person to "be happy", you can't tell a procrastinator to "just do it!" It's completely disrespectful and often not realistic.

It's also the reason I get a little nervous writing this book. There is no one-size-fits-all solution to procrastination. Every person's experience is something different and there may be a genuine medical reason underlying someone's tendency to put things off and struggle to self-motivate. There are also some more modern suggestions that we stall on our actions because we are more likely to follow our natural impulses to do things that excite us. Our modern day living allows us easy and fast access to so many things in an instant. This causes our brain's nerve cells to release dopamine to other nerve cells creating a neural pathway. Dopamine is released when your brain is expecting a reward. It helps motivate you to take action. The problem in our contemporary way of living is we are bombarded by constant dopamine hits as we pull towards the need and desire for immediate reward. That's why it's so hard to resist checking Instagram, Twitter and Facebook. You can be rewarded with a delicious carb, fat and sugar filled meal within minutes of ordering it at your local fast food restaurant. We can fake our natural sexual impulses of dopamine and oxytocin by glimpsing into the sexual activity of strangers through watching porn. Even the ping of an incoming email has the power to release dopamine and cause us to spend an additional estimated 23 minutes getting back into our focused work[6]. Our new fast world means faster impulses, an increase in dopamine surges resulting in changing the way our brains work.

Brain trauma, depression, anxiety, low self esteem or dopamine overload aside, we have all experienced procrastination in some form. World renowned psychologist Sigmund Freud concluded that people have the instinctive desire to act in a way that sees us seek out pleasure and avoid pain to satisfy biological and psychological needs[7]. We are hard wired as human beings to look for the pleasurable things in life and avoid the stuff that sucks. Great analysis, but that doesn't help us when our livelihood and ability to pay the mortgage depends on our performance at work which is completely dependent on our productivity.

So what can we do about procrastination if we don't have brain trauma, illness or medication blocking our natural ability to get things done?

Overcoming procrastination is often a journey of learning to trust yourself again. We make these promises to ourselves that we'll take action, or get things done by a certain day and time but what happens? We don't do it. We become distracted and because of this, things are left unfinished. What happens to our inner psyche when we do this repeatedly? Trust in ourselves is lost and if we can't trust ourselves, who can? This mistrust snowballs into feelings of disappointment, sadness and failure. This is such a shame as it is relatively easy to overcome - if we take rapid action that doesn't allow us to overthink it!

The answer to your own procrastinating tendencies is down to you to find out. I've been on my own mission to find out what works for me, my clients and others and I've collated these fantastic ways in order to help you view procrastination differently and create your own toolkit that 'future you' will thank you for.

I wanted to write this book in a certain way that could be referred back to, time and time again. I wanted to incorporate as many strategies as I could find, along with the science or tried and tested experience behind it to hopefully give fellow procrastinators something they can turn to quickly that might help inspire them into action.

What type of procrastinator are you?

I came across this great article written by Darren Tong, the co-editor of Alpha Efficiency magazine. Darren suggests that we each usually fit into the following four procrastination categories[8];

1. Anxious procrastination
2. Fun procrastination
3. "Plenty of time" procrastination
4. Perfectionist procrastination

Anxious procrastination

This presents as anxiety around getting started and completing any task or decision. Anxiety procrastination is when you worry about the time it will take or the action, resources and knowledge needed to get the task done.

Worrying about the future implications associated with the task can put you in an anxiety loop. For example, students who want to achieve good grades think too far ahead into the future and the enormity of the exams causes anxiety. They know they need the grades to get to college, to get the good job, get the house, get the family and 2.4 kids and all of a sudden their whole life is riding on those exams. While this can sometimes be a natural motivator to achieve good grades, it often feels so huge that the person will respond with anxious thoughts and completely stall even starting their studies.

This might also present when training for a big sporting race, going for that job promotion, new job or attempting to lose a large amount of weight. You might be able to visualise 'future you' but you focus so much on the current gap between 'present you' and 'future you' that your anxiety spikes. You feel so far away from that future person you know you want to become. It seems like too huge a task to get there and achieve the dream goal, it feels impossible. What happens? Your anxiety chooses to stay safe as 'present you' and doesn't take any action or makes little progress. That's why visualisation and breaking down the steps into manageable chunks can help progression.

Fun procrastination

The fun procrastinator hates doing the boring stuff. They like to be happy and comfortable and go for instant gratification over delayed reward.

Why eat a salad when a pizza is so much more delicious?

Why start that paper when you can watch TV?

Why go out for a run when you can play video games?

What may seem like fun at the time soon turns into stress when the inevitable task needs to be completed anyway. The fun procrastinators benefit from 'active' procrastination and scheduling in the fun stuff first into their diaries. Equally, focusing on the fun stuff they like to procrastinate on as a form of a reward can help too. Making productivity fun helps the fun procrastinator too. I identify with this type of procrastination when I'm trying to write. So I make my writing environment and process as fun as possible. We'll cover more on this in the chapters around music anchoring, factoring in play, setting the right environment and creating a reward system.

'Plenty of time' procrastination

This is the procrastinator who knows a task is due but it is a long way off. "I've got plenty of time" they think to themselves. Yet deadline day approaches and it's all panic stations as they struggle to get their tasks finished. Students are classic 'plenty of time' procrastinators. Their final papers are due at the end of the year. They're supposed to put a whole academic year of study into the paper but what happens? A week to go and they're pulling all nighters trying to cram a year's worth of study into 100 hours of poor work.

Many journalists naturally work in this way. Being used to strict, hard and final deadlines on print or going on air, journalists are deadline driven creatures. Articles are moved, news items are brought forward or breaking news happens and it is all systems go. It is an industry that thrives on positive and exciting stress. The adrenaline rush of making the evening papers or being the first with an exclusive comes in handy when those other longer deadline pieces are suddenly and unexpectedly due.

'Plenty of time' procrastination can present in our inability to save money for the future or even pay into a pension fund. Our retirement seems so far away so why put money away right now in the prime of life? How many of us put off siphoning money away for our tax returns and then struggle to make the payment at the end of the financial year?

There's joy in the cumulative effect of small action and not putting things off. A good example of this is the penny challenge. Many banks can automate this process for you where they automatically save a penny (one cent) on day one, two pence (two cents) on day two, three pence on day three until day 365 and £3.65 ($3.65) is transferred into a separate savings account. At the end of the year you will have saved almost £700 ($700) by doing nothing at all!

One way to help the 'plenty of time' style of procrastination is to go public or get accountability to support you to achieve your goal. We'll cover this in the chapters about accountability, getting help and changing the deadlines.

Perfectionist procrastination

If you have a perfectionist type personality, your own need for everything to be perfect can stop you in your tracks before you've even started. Perfectionists spend a lot of time thinking about how to make everything perfect. They might be exceptional planners and strategists but not great implementers.

A fear of failure or not being good enough keeps a perfectionist in the procrastination zone. A hard deadline puts a perfectionist into a corner and they have no choice but to take action. That action might be sub-standard to what they originally envisioned in their view of a 'perfect' outcome which causes stress at the completion of a task.

The chapters around perfectionism, keeping a win list, being enough, the fear list and the F*ck-it Bucket are all excellent coping strategies for the perfectionists among us.

Chapter 2

Drop the Perfectionism

Affirmation: Life is never truly perfect but I am perfectly capable of creating a truly great life.

Journal prompt: What does perfect look like? Does it exist? Explain.

*

Having continually high standards is inherent in modern day society. We are constantly expected to improve and exceed expectations from childhood through to retirement. We are assessed and evaluated through every stage of our lives and expected to do better. In our education and jobs, our performance is assessed. We are expected to achieve more and more. In sales, we are always asked to make more money year on year, our targets do not decrease.

In a society where everyone and every stage of our lives demands more, is it any wonder we get bogged down and overwhelmed with the need to keep being better, doing better and becoming perfect?

Perfectionism is one of the most debilitating forms of procrastination. The two go hand in hand playing a merry dance that keeps people stuck. Steeped in low self esteem, perfectionism sees someone paralysed by the fear of failure and not being good enough - so they either waste valuable time trying to make everything perfect before taking action or take no action at all.

Perfectionism is such a toxic trait because it can be so negative. A perfectionist desires success more than anything. Before taking any form of action, a perfectionist has already decided what success looks like, instead of making a start, propelling forwards and tweaking as they go.

We've seen a rise in perfectionism in the last 30 years. It isn't just the average parents wanting the best for their children, pushing us to achieve, achieve, achieve. We know that social media and comparison of others plays a part in the perfectionism/procrastination cycle. In the past, we didn't know what other people did and in such detail like we do now with social media. We are offered a daily, sometimes hourly glimpse into people's lives and it causes us to feel like a failure as the voyeurs of the filtered lives of others. We see people achieving their goals and we often don't feel the same.

Hewitt and Flett's 45-item Multidimensional Perfectionism Scale (MPS; Hewitt & Flett, 1991, 2004)[1] is a widely-used instrument to assess the different types of perfectionism according to the Perfectionism Scale. Their research highlighted the different forms of perfectionism to be aware of:

- Self-oriented perfectionism is where the person cannot progress until imposing their own unrealistic levels of perfectionism on themselves. A self-oriented perfectionist will adhere to strict standards while maintaining strong motivation to attain perfection and avoid failure.

- Other-oriented perfectionism is where a person will impose their own unrealistic standards of perfection on others. An other-oriented perfectionist will set unrealistic standards for significant others (e.g., partners, children, co-workers) coupled with a stringent evaluation of others' performances.

- Socially prescribed perfectionism is where a person will expect unrealistic perfection from others. Socially prescribed perfectionists believe that others hold unrealistic expectations for their behaviour (and that they can't live up to this). They experience external pressure to be perfect and believe others evaluate them critically.

There are other research papers that research the positive and negative traits of perfectionism. I suggest reading Andrews, D. M., Burns, L. R., & Dueling, J. K. (2014). Positive perfectionism: Seeking the healthy "should", or should we?. Open Journal of Social Sciences, 2(08), 27.[2]

Although not included in Hewitt and Flett's Multidimensional Perfectionism Scale, all perfectionism isn't bad so I'd like to include this one;

- Positive perfectionism is where a person has diligence, a conscientious approach, inner self discipline and positively utilises perfectionism to make headway on their goals. Otherwise known as being consistently conscientious.

I know a couple of people in my own life that would identify as positive perfectionists. This book is not for them or others who are also able to be consistently conscientious.

Perfectionism in action in our lives

The workplace is a common breeding ground for perfectionism in action. Employees are driven and judged by their performance, often not able to differentiate between their work and a personal and emotive subject. People questioned about the quality of their work can feel attacked. If this has happened once before, an employee might find themselves completely stuck and plagued by procrastination because they don't want to mess up. They're concerned about the evaluation of their work by others.

You may have experienced this yourself, depending on the type of work you have experienced. In this corporate scenario, you submit work to a superior and then as the email reply pings in your inbox, your heart sinks as you automatically fear the worst and tell yourself it isn't good enough. Or worse still, you submit work to a superior and get no feedback at all causing anxiety around the next task or report you have to submit.

You might have even experienced a scenario where a once generous deadline actually gave you too much time to think and perfect a pitch, presentation or report. You got the brief weeks ago and were so enthusiastic and full of ideas - this was your chance to make it absolutely water tight and flawless! So you read more, researched more and before you knew it, you found yourself in an endless Google scroll going from one topic to the other just wasting time trying to ensure your work is exemplary. You've wasted so much time on it, or wasted so much mental energy just thinking about it and not taking action, that you're now hours away from the deadline and flooded with adrenaline, anxiety and stress to get it finished - never mind perfect.

In professions where competition between colleagues is high on the agenda, perfectionism can manifest as a direct response to fear of failing against a colleague. A perfectionist might stall on their daily tasks due to a fear of criticism from colleagues or superiors on the quality of their work. In professions where team members rely on the progression of tasks with many employees involved in the process, a perfectionist may slow down or completely block the chain of work for fear of judgement on their part of the process. We all know someone who wants something to be "top notch" or "just right" and we get frustrated at their painfully slow working speed as they spend far too much time on their tasks and delay everyone else in the process.

Another example of self-oriented perfectionism, but away from the workplace, might be the desire to make a lifestyle change. Someone may look at pictures on Instagram of others who have overhauled their lives and thought "I want that too". They took up a sport, changed what they ate and in turn changed how they looked, thought, and felt. Yet they see others living a 'perfect' life and cannot see themselves doing the same. Perfect seems too much and too unattainable.

There are countless people who desperately want to make a change to their lives, but they don't ever start. The secret to making a lasting lifestyle change is to take it slow and steady and change one thing at a time; an extra litre of water tomorrow, saying no to those cakes the day after, increasing their daily steps over the course of a week. All of these small action steps, like compound interest, build over time to create great results. Yet many people think they need to change everything in one day in order to be healthy. They know they might need to avoid junk food, head to the gym three times a week and cut down on the alcohol consumption but focusing on all of those actions at once makes it feel too much. Being 'perfect' is too far out of their comfort zone so they do nothing. They keep scrolling on their phones on social media, feeling crap about themselves instead of making the smallest change and making it consistently until it is a habit. You will never hate yourself into being happy. You will never make a change that sticks and becomes a habit if you try to change too many things at once.

What is the cost of perfectionism?

Psychologists agree that there are many positive and negative aspects of perfectionism[3]. For the person who is able to use perfectionism alongside self discipline they will continue to take action, make progress and produce thorough results. These people who are able to blend the two and who seem to have willpower of steel are definitely in the minority. They're the ones who get the report submitted with days to spare. They're the people who get up early and go to the gym every morning. They're the ones who can diligently work on a book or a project every day for months and be ready ahead of their self imposed deadline. They're not the people this book was written for!

The majority of us with perfectionism tendencies sees us attempting to achieve unattainable goals or setting unrealistic deadlines for ourselves. This can often lead to depression and low self esteem caused by feeling like a repeated failure when you cannot live up to your own unfeasible ideals.

I know this manifested for me with my clients. I would tell people I would have work completed by certain dates and then just stall, without taking any action. I'd think about it. A lot. I'd be walking the dog or cleaning up and it would be in my mind constantly on how to make it perfect, yet I couldn't take action or that first step to just sit down and start. I feared I was terrible at my job and wasn't good enough. This was the subliminal message I sent to my subconscious and my mindset responded by keeping me stuck in procrastination but with that perfectionism blocking me from making one single step into action.

How do we get over it?

Learn to get better at being worse

I know, that sounds insane right? However, done or started is better than perfect and stalled. We have to get good as we go along, but we have to get started first. So learning to get better at being worse is the key.

Have a conversation with yourself, a trusted friend or loved one. Get honest about what your perfectionism is costing you personally in terms of your productivity and stress levels.

Open up the chat and discuss what perfect actually looks like. Is it real? Is it attainable? Do you have the time, talent and drive to make whatever it is you're focusing on perfect? What will suffice and be a good job, rather than a perfect one? How will you get there to achieve OK and satisfactory? What will the benefits be to you personally if you're able to finish tasks quicker? Or if it is a lifestyle change, what small actions could you build on and focus on first?

Choose between punishment vs praise and reward

Think about your own perfectionism. In the past have you ever been rewarded or punished when you strived to be perfect? If you tried to do well at school, worked hard to improve and be 'perfect,' what happened? Were you praised by teachers and parents? Did you receive treats and rewards for a job well done?

Now think about your perfectionism as punishment. Where have your perfectionist tendencies caused you to be punished? Have you been chastised by a superior at work, or a teacher, or a parent in the past? Have you punished yourself for your perfectionism? Have you ended up staying awake all night, causing untold stress and sleep deprivation trying to get your tasks completed by the unrealistic deadline?

Ask yourself which feels better?

It's quite sad to realise that from the moment we are born we are on an expected path of constant improvement. This is life. This is what we have been born into and we can't change it. The good news is we are capable of changing the stress we put ourselves under as we naturally fight back against it.

So next time you find yourself stalled and stuck because you're overthinking tasks, taking too long, trying to get it perfect and procrastinating, ask yourself what it would feel like to get it done and be praised and rewarded. Even if that is self reward. When you make promises to yourself and keep them, that is very powerful. So break down that next task, set realistic deadlines and appointments with yourself to get it completed (done is better than perfect remember) and focus on the praise and reward at the end - even if both come from yourself!

Be honest about your fear of judgement

Who is judging you? Who is expecting you to be better and who might critique your work or efforts? Have you actually ever asked these people what they really think? Have you asked for their help or even their feedback on how you could stop stressing so much about making everything perfect?

Your perfectionism is probably linked to your fear of criticism, judgement and the fear of other people thinking you have failed. If you tell yourself enough times that you're no good at something and are a failure you'll act in that same way. When you act in that same way, you become who you tell yourself you are.

So judging yourself also comes into this. What impossible standards and rules are you imposing on yourself? Where have they come from? What will it mean if you drop your standards slightly? What will it mean if you set more realistic expectations and stick to your promises?

Place a temporary ban on technology

In a new digital age it is the overwhelm of information that often keeps us stuck in perfection. If you're writing a report, creating a presentation or like me right now, writing a book why not impose a technology ban? Turn off the internet for a set period of time (I'm going for a 25 minute Pomodoro device-free session as I type this). I have done this right now because I found myself getting overwhelmed and bogged down in the research. I've just read three scientific papers and have been doing that annoying thing where you absentmindedly click from one link to another to another. The truth is I've been researching this chapter for a month and I know what I want to say. This book is not a book on perfectionism, it is a book on overcoming procrastination and while perfectionism is a big part of that, it isn't the whole book. So the internet is now turned off while I refer to my hand written research and type out this chapter.

If you would like to read these studies on overcoming perfectionism in more depth, please search for 'Riley et al 2007 Perfectionism'[4] to read the paper and associated studies that outline different therapies that were successfully utilised in reducing perfectionism in participants.

Actively reduce your expectation on yourself and others

Constantly expecting others and yourself to behave in a certain way is not healthy or productive. While we are the only people in control of our thoughts and behaviours, placing too many unrealistic goals on ourselves and having high expectations could cause us emotional pain. It is the same for our expectations of others. Often if we place high expectations on ourselves, we will also do this with those around us. Nobody is perfect. Nobody is a mind reader. While you can't force anyone to behave in a way that pleases you, if you need people to be a certain way, ask for what you want and need. You can ask for support and help. If you just expect it to magically happen, you may end up feeling disappointed. If you expect too much and place tight time restrictions on yourself, you may be destined to fail. So ask where you are expecting too much from yourself and others? How is it having a negative impact in your life?

Get help for social anxiety

In the Riley et al 2007 Perfectionism study referenced above, Cognitive Behavioural Therapy (CBT) was successfully utilised to treat social anxiety which in turn reduced levels of perfectionism. If you are someone who is suffering from what could be deemed as clinical perfectionism, particularly around eating disorders and debilitating perfectionism that is causing stress, anxiety and depression then therapy could be a positive route. A CBT therapist will be able to point out where your beliefs around being perfect have started and help you forge a new positive path to reducing perfectionism in your life.

Chapter 3

Count Down and Take Action

Affirmation: I am capable of making important decisions in an instant.

Journal Prompt: Change happens in an instant with an instant decision. Think back to when you have decided to make a change in a split second decision. How did it work out? What did it lead to? What did you go on to achieve after you made that decision?

*

I'll start the procrastination busting tips with this one because it's the simplest and easiest when trying to take action. It's so easy, even a toddler could do it.

Have you come across the best selling book The 5 Second Rule[1] by international speaker and author, Mel Robbins?

If you haven't read the book allow me to summarise;

Procrastinating on something? Count down 5..4..3..2..1 and TAKE ACTION!

That's it. It's that simple. That's the book!

Isn't it true that any decision in our lives is this simple? Yes or no. Start or don't. Finish it or leave it. We often regularly choose to make it more complicated than it needs to be.

If 5…4…3…2…1… was that easy any smoker could give up a lifetime of cigarette smoking in five seconds. Any unfit wannabe athlete could head out and run a marathon. Any competent swimmer could head out to swim a mile. Yet our brain often blocks this simplicity and gives us excuses and barriers to why we can't take action. We think of the pain or the restriction or the suffering that could possibly happen if we just got on with it. We think about the consequences too much and before you know it we are in a spiral of procrastinating again.

How many times throughout your life have you used the counting down technique to drown out those fears of the consequences and just take action?

What about the times you've counted to 10 to calm down?

Or the times you've counted down from five when trying to discipline your kids or your pets?

Have you ever counted to three and then just jumped into a potentially freezing swimming pool?

We count down because it helps us to focus on the task in hand and take action quickly. Counting down doesn't give us time to consider the external factors and consequences that might happen once we jump in.

Mel Robbins came up with the idea of the 5 Second Rule many years ago. The life that she and her husband were both leading was stressful and causing her to feel low and helpless. She was unemployed, in financial trouble, consuming too much alcohol to numb her stress and she felt like she wasn't being a very good parent or wife. Her husband was also going through some career difficulties and they both felt like they existed in a sea of permanent stress. Neither of them were taking much action to get on top of their situation and improve their circumstances.

One evening while watching TV, Mel spotted an advertisement which featured a rocket launch. What happens at all rocket launches? We're shown NASA employees both in mission control and the astronauts on board the rocket. Everyone is filled with anticipation, all waiting on the big momentous countdown of "5..4..3..2..1…and we have lift off!" It is a phrase that is ingrained in our minds whenever we think of space exploration and one sentence that has become part of our modern vocabulary when talking about taking action.

Mel watched this commercial and noted to herself that she needed more of the '5…4…3…2…1 lift off!' in her own life to get motivated to make positive changes. She decided to put this to the test the very next morning. On going to bed, she made a promise to herself that when her alarm sounded she would think 5…4…3…2…1.. get up! The next morning she did just this. Instead of lazing in bed and snoozing the alarm multiple times she got straight up and started her day. This one small action became life changing for her as she started to implement this simple counting down trick for many moments, decisions and actions in her life.

So why is counting down so simple and effective?

Mel explains in her book, The 5 Second Rule, that if you "have an impulse to act on a goal you must physically move within 5 seconds or your brain will kill the idea." You've probably experienced this for yourself in the past. You've got ready to go for a run but come to lace your sneakers on and think "Oh I can't be bothered." Nonetheless, you've overridden those thoughts of staying in your comfort zone and not just put on those sneakers but you've headed out of the door to run too. Physically moving is powerful and doesn't allow too much inner conflict with your brain which has the potential to talk you out of action.

The more you do it, the more courageous you will become

The repeated habit of using the 5 second rule to take action makes you less afraid to make a start over time. It will help you strengthen those productivity muscles as you fire into gear quicker than your subconscious can shift you into reverse.

Every time you use the 5 second rule, it is an act of courage. You are fighting back against your comfort zone and your worst enemy - your inner negative voice. From each small act of courage, more courage follows. The more you implement the 5 second rule, the more you create a compound effect of courageous positive change. The more you build on that compound effect, the more you trust yourself again.

What happens when you trust yourself? You know you have it in you to take action and achieve all you are capable of. There is nothing more disheartening than knowing you have amazing potential but you're just not able to knuckle down and act on it.

There is never a right time so stop wasting time and start

"The diet starts Monday" is something I'm sure we've all thought or said aloud in our lifetime. Why do we wait for a new week for a new start? Why can't we start right now? The answer is because we are ALWAYS looking for the right time for everything in our lives. That's why we continually put things off, waiting for the right point to start.

In my day to day life of marketing and copywriting I work closely with a number of fitness professionals. These personal trainers and fitness specialists work with people across all walks of life to support them to achieve their fat loss and muscle building goals. One thing that always struck me when working in this sector is the time it takes for a potential new client to finally make contact and get the help they know they need. The number of people who have the means to invest but delay taking action to employ the services of these fitness professionals astounds me. They wait for a new job, new month, landmark birthday or to move house or the kids to go back to school FIRST before getting started. The ironic thing is that these stressful life situations are easier to manage when you're looking after your health and well-being but people continuously put it off until they feel the time is right.

Then they achieve their goals, have an awesome before and after picture and we interview them for a testimonial. What's the ONE thing they ALL say? "I wish I'd started sooner". Facepalm moment or what?

We all have to go through a bit of mental pain to change the physical and emotional pain that keeps us stuck. It is part and parcel of transformation. Make these decisions to take action repeatedly and it becomes easier and easier.

Once we decide we want to change our lives we have two choices; we can take immediate action or we can sit daydreaming about the right time to start, the actions we will take and what the end will look like. We wait for change to just magically happen and keep ourselves stuck by waiting for that right moment to occur. Often we decide to make a change once we are in a place of so much pain that the only option is to make a change and make it immediately. But why wait until that distressing point of emotional pain to make a change? Wouldn't it be kinder on yourself and your nervous system to decide to make a change from a place of positivity rather than desperation?

Change is always new. It is always uncertain. It is always tinged with a sense of fear. This is all completely normal but you can overcome it and make the art of change become a valuable part of your new comfort zone. You can get to grips with change, learn to love it and see it as a positive step for self-growth.

It doesn't matter whether you have a fitness or fat loss goal, whether you want to get your finances in order, whether you want to grow your business or improve your love life - all these require change and you can either sit on your ass waiting for them to appear, or you can take small repeated actions right now. Waiting and sitting on this inevitable need for action is prolonging your pain and it is causing you to mistrust the only person you can truly rely on - yourself!

The five second rule is a psychological intervention

When you're using this quick fire technique to shift you from procrastination to productivity, you are overriding your feelings and emotions, which in turn makes you more resilient.

This is an example of a psychological intervention in action. As our feelings are just suggestions, using psychological intervention helps us override these feelings.

In the book Descartes' Error, world famous neuroscientist Antonio Damasio compiled research to suggest that as much as 95% of our decisions every day are decided by our feelings rather than facts[2]. Damasio referred to us human beings as "Feeling machines that think, not thinking machines that feel". So our usual scenario is to feel then think, rather than the other way around. So we feel, think and then act!

Knowing this is how we operate as human beings, why do we procrastinate? Because we feel like we can't do it, can't be bothered, are not good enough etc. Rather than thinking we can't do it. We momentarily feel the pain of productivity and therefore then think "Nope!" putting a stop to our actions. Have you ever wanted to run or set a goal to run? What happened? Your brain felt the pain of the run on your feet, the tightness in your chest and the pressure on your lungs and felt like it could be too painful and difficult, therefore making you think you couldn't do it or didn't want to do it. The result? You acted on that thought that came from the feeling and you didn't run. If you have ever done the opposite and pushed through this feeling to go run, swim or cycle anyway then you've proved that you can override these feelings that lead to the thoughts which lead to procrastination.

Use 5…4…3…2…1…GO as an instant solution to procrastination. It is a bona fide psychological intervention that overrides your subconscious talking you out of taking action. Do it often enough and you strengthen your mental resolve, easily catapulting yourself right forwards into the act of taking action.

Have you read enough already and you're ready to take action? Think about that one thing you've been procrastinating on and the first step you need to take to get it done. Say the following out loud:

5…4…3…2…1…GO! And do it!

Chapter 4

The Two Minute Rule for Getting Things Done

Affirmation: I can reach any goal, one tiny step at a time.

Journal Prompt: Thinking about the one thing you have been procrastinating on recently, what is the very first step that you could do in under two minutes to get you started?

*

The last chapter explored the Five Second Rule as a method to make a rapid decision and spring into action. Sometimes we might need just a little longer to get our feet off the starting blocks. Most of our desired accomplishments can be achieved when we break each step down to the most granular detail.

Imagine a big goal you might have. It could be running a marathon or writing a book. This big goal will only be achieved by repeated small consistent actions that lead to success and accomplishing the overall objective. When we set our hearts on these goals the hardest part is remaining consistent with our actions in order to achieve what we set out to do. That's why creating a goal habit using a two minute rule could really assist you in getting into the routine of positive consistent action.

Take the example of running a marathon. Could you run a marathon tomorrow? Possibly.

Even with no training under your belt you could just decide to head out there and go for it. It might take you a full day, you might make lots of stops, your feet might end up blistered and you could end up injured but you also could do it. However, that would be very painful and very hard. You'd need a mindset of steel to push through the physical, emotional and mental pain to get to the finish.

That's why the majority of people running a marathon will follow a training programme months in advance. They'll break down their running into smaller, more manageable goals and each week build on the progress of the previous week until they're running 20+ miles just a fortnight before the race. I'm part of a running team and there are a small number of the team who have places at this year's London Marathon. We have a WhatsApp group chat and this morning they have been sending us updates on their 16 mile run they completed today. It has been so inspirational to watch these weekly updates and the mileage increasing each week as they follow their training programme. There are just eight weeks to go until the London Marathon and they are feeling confident and prepared. I adore following their progress as they're an example of consistent action, repeated over time, which is building their habits, expertise, strength and stamina.

This time last year if you had told our novice runners that they would be running a marathon they would not have believed you. Because even getting to the point of running regularly is the hard part here. Our brains want to keep us in our comfort zone and heading out to pound the streets and spending hours in training running miles in preparation for a marathon is the most difficult part of this process. When the first run has been hellish, how do you keep your motivation to go back and repeat it until you improve?

That's where the two minute rule comes in.

Instead of setting a goal of say running 50 miles a week which can completely freak a novice runner out, take it back down to the very basics and decide what would take less than two minutes and get you into the right physical state to start training.

Examples of two minute tasks that would set you up to run:

- Getting your gym bag ready and packed in the car three times a week
- Lacing up your trainers
- Listening to a motivational running song

The trick is to decide on one thing, then set THAT as your goal. Let's use the example of lacing up your trainers. Instead of saying you will run 50 miles per week, tell yourself you will change into your running clothes and lace up your trainers three times a week. Decide which days and times in the week this will happen. Stick a reminder in your calendar. Remind yourself you're just lacing up and tying your trainers.

This one small two minute action will be the catalyst to start running. Once you start running you're on your way to achieving your goal of training for and then running a marathon. It will help you build your running habit and help you overcome your subconscious that is always trying to keep you in your comfort zone.

I can tell you from experience that when you decide to run a marathon, if you're not an experienced runner the thought of 26.2 miles is almost nauseating. I can't quite believe it but I have completed the London Marathon twice. Sadly, I did not train properly either time and I found the whole experience a nightmare, to say the least. I sat at home and thought about running, dreading it until it got to about eight weeks before the race and I decided I really should put in some training effort. This is a typical example of someone only acting at that critical point of emergency to get something done.

I can look back on my own marathon experience and realise I was completely overwhelmed at the thought of the mileage. I sat stressing about it instead of taking action. I didn't build any habits around training and therefore set myself up to fail. Even though I completed the race twice, it was very painful and I caused myself more harm than good by entering into it unprepared. Which is why I love seeing my running team mates putting in such stellar effort every week to follow their training programme to the letter. I know their marathon experience will be much more enjoyable than mine.

Let's review the other example above of setting a goal of writing a book. As an author myself and regularly interviewing authors on my BBC Radio show, writing a book is something the general public find very impressive. I know when I wrote my first book, Self Discipline: A How-to Guide to Stop Procrastinating and Achieve Your Goals[1], I was shocked how many people were genuinely taken aback that I'd written a book. A little like a marathon, it is something people deem as very difficult, arduous and lengthy.

Interviewing other authors has revealed that many of us procrastinate on actually sitting down to write, which obviously is the first step to doing anything! If we can't sit down to write, we can't possibly finish a book.

So the two minute rule on writing might be:

- sitting down at your desk to write
- setting a timer to write
- opening up a writing app or Word

Each of these examples above might take a lot less time than two minutes, seconds even. It is about putting you in the right state to make a start. I've done the above three things myself in this writing session right now as I write this chapter. I put it in my diary last week that I would be writing at this time (and told my accountability buddy I would check in with them after writing). I have made the right writing environment for me at my desk with candles lit, blanket round my shoulders, binaural beats playing on my headphones and coffee to my right. I've set a 25 minute timer to write as part of my Pomodoro process (see Chapter 8 for more on this) and I've opened Ulysses writing app. Setting an intention of 'Make coffee, light a candle, play binaural beats and open Ulysses' five times a week feels a lot less overwhelming than 'Write 20,000 words this week' or 'Write a book'. It's been broken down and my brain can compute that it is manageable.

If you think about your own big goals, what could you do in two minutes that is going to get you in the right mindset to start? Break it down into two minutes to make it achievable. Any of us can commit to a simple two minute action. Keeping things to two minutes and then following through with your required actions will, over time, add up to success with your big goals.

The two minute rule for getting things done

We have the two minute rule for breaking down tasks, but there's also a well known two minute rule for clearing the annoyingly mundane tasks that threaten to take up too much valuable brain space. It is a way to stop distracting thoughts and 'to-do' items from building and adding up to one huge backlog of things you need to do.

Addressing two minute tasks immediately

David Allen, a leading management consultant and productivity expert authored the world famous Getting Things Done: The Art of Stress Free Productivity[2]. He is renowned for his methods that help companies move their goals forwards by focusing on the action taking habits of those at an executive level. David Allen has many celebrated methods in his system for productivity but the two minute rule is one that always stands out.

How many different incoming demands happen to you each day that would take two minutes or less? On a personal level it might be clearing away your plate after dinner, taking the household garbage out, or putting a washing load on. It could be wiping down the shower screen after you've washed, folding some laundry or feeding the dog. Each of these tasks take two minutes or less but we often will completely avoid them, put them off and then what? They build until we get to a point of emergency where we feel like we have so much to do to 'get straight' and clear the decks on these tasks. If we had tackled these small tasks as we went about our day they'd be sorted, completed and we wouldn't be wasting our precious brain space stressing about them.

It's the same in an office environment. There might be an email, a phone call, a conversation with a colleague that needs to happen in order to progress a project. Yet we add these things onto our ever growing to-do list instead of tackling it right there and then. These will all waste time later as we review and organise them instead of just getting it done.

David Allen believes that if there is an incoming task that will take two minutes or less, DO IT NOW. Get it done so you do not then think about it twice, three times or even five times. This is a waste of energy and thinking space. Get things done and get them down now.

While I am recommending two minutes as a rule for clearing the decks, there are some that argue the two minute time limit has its flaws. If the tasks you can think of that come to mind might take longer than two minutes, read on to the next chapter for what might be a better solution for you.

Chapter 5

The Five Minute Rule - More Realistic Than Two Minutes?

Affirmation: Time is on my side. I can achieve everything I desire quickly and easily.

Journal Prompt: What can I achieve today in less than five minutes that my future self will thank me for?

*

Could five minutes be better than two?

In the previous chapter we covered both sides of the coin for the two minute rule. One side is offered as a way to build goal habits for larger goals and reduce overwhelm. The other side of the two minute rule advises clearing anything that takes two minutes or less immediately in order to stop wasting precious thinking time dealing with it later.

But is two minutes realistic? Does it give you enough time?

This is the counter argument for the two minute rule which is why I'm including this chapter on increasing that same concept to five minutes.

Mike Vardy from Productivityist argues that two minute tasks don't always work[1]. That call you wanted to make to a client, that email you needed to send to a co-worker might go from a two minute task to a 30 minute "time sucking vampire" which could ultimately completely derail your productivity and progress for the day. If you have ever tried clearing incoming tasks as soon as they arrive, you might have experienced this yourself. What you hoped would only take minutes can end up leeching your time.

As with any productivity method, it takes time to fully audit yourself and your own circumstances. How you work best, what your office environment is like, your daily distractions, your own personal responsibilities and other variables like the others you rely on in order to complete your work is different for each person. I am four years into my own quest for ultimate productivity and even though I feel like I have completely nailed it when it comes to sitting down and being focused, there are so many different factors that stand in my way and put the brakes on every single day.

We know that getting back into focused work takes around 20 minutes after each disruption. So is addressing two minute tasks as they arrive in your inbox, to your phone or via a verbal command the right method for you? Or will this completely disrupt and displace your day?

You know yourself better than anyone. You know which parts of your life you always seem to procrastinate on. So if you think you can get things done and off your list and out of your head in two minutes then great! Adopt the two minute method. Yet if your own circumstances mean that two minutes isn't realistic then could you increase it to five minutes?

Also is two minutes a clunky time that has the potential to easily run over? David Allen, author of Getting Things Done advises the executives he coaches to have a good 30-90 minutes every morning free of meetings to work on two minute tasks. This seems to contradict the other advice of actioning the tasks as they arrive. Also 30-90 minutes seems like a long time and would mean the average executive working on 15-45 tiny tasks. Is this achievable? Or would each one run over therefore causing more overwhelm?

I am a huge fan of the Pomodoro technique for productivity (see chapter 8) because this method naturally allows a five minute break, I have found from my own experience that I use this five minute period to focus on the small tasks and get them off my list. I work for 25 minutes without distractions so no phone, email and ideally no other person to interrupt.

When the five minute rest timer sounds I will take my phone and make a drink, use the bathroom, walk to chat to a colleague if I am working in a client's business - whatever is needed to do. I'll try to reply to messages and emails while the coffee brews. I might use the five minutes if I'm working from home to put a laundry load on, feed the dogs, or call my husband. Then as soon as the timer sounds, I'm back at my desk ready to work in the next 25 minute chunk.

From personal experience I have found that five minutes works better for me. When I think I have two minutes, for a start, this didn't fit in with my Pomodoro timer anyway. This allowed for 2.5 two minute tasks and they ALWAYS ran over. I had a tendency to try and achieve too much in that time, whereas focusing on five minutes seems more manageable.

I also started to notice how long things took. I wrote about this in my last book. I went on a little conscious timing spree to see how long things actually took me. I was shocked that the most common household tasks I always seemed to procrastinate on took such a small amount of time. Things like making my bed took 30 seconds, putting the dishes away took three minutes, putting a load of laundry in the tumble dryer took 50 seconds and changing the toilet paper took 10 seconds. Yet I still wasn't doing these simple tasks as and when they cropped up.

When I increased my time limit for addressing these menial jobs that were regularly building and causing future stress, I found a solution. Giving myself a five minute break in my Pomodoro timed tasks allowed me to factor in a quick audit of rooms in the house. For example, on a five minute break I might schedule a quick tidy up around the living room. I work at speed doing this (it's become a weird but fun game to me) and as the five minute timer goes off I will plump the sofa cushions, clear clutter, or maybe whip the vacuum cleaner round or dust the TV. I might not have realised all that needed doing and as far as the two minute rule goes - these aren't necessarily incoming tasks, but I definitely feel the cumulative effect of working this way when at the end of the day my work is complete and the house is in a semi-decent clean and tidy state.

Obviously this only works if you work from home like me, but in your five minute break at work you could still get tasks marked off. That email that needs sending, the call to a client, the quick question you need to ask your team. All these smaller tasks are often the precursor and next step to moving larger tasks along. Even taking five minutes away from your monitor and going for a short walk or taking some conscious deep breaths all helps break up the day and allows you to refocus.

If you're at home relaxing and watching mainstream TV then the commercial breaks also act as a good five minute pause to get smaller jobs done. When I used to work on the radio in a team on the breakfast show, when the commercials were playing my producer and I would do press ups, sit ups or jog on the spot. We made a big joke about it on air at the time but we carried on for months. It made a massive difference to our physique and strength and complemented our gym routines and runs. I know my cousin does repeated squats by the bathroom sink every time she brushes her teeth. Twice a day, every day, without fail.

I have a friend who works in finance and she uses a daily five minute break to record her receipts and financial transactions, check her bank statement and 'skim' save money. This is where you check your balance and round it down to a numerical figure of your choice. For example, if her bank statement says £357.80 she has decided to round it down to the nearest zero so transfers £7.80 into her savings leaving the balance at a rounded £350. It only takes her five minutes every day but her financial spreadsheets are always up to date and she saves a lot of money. Do this yourself daily and you'll soon accrue a healthy savings account.

There's no right answer whether you commit to two minute tasks or five minute tasks. You know yourself which will work best for you. Try implementing this five minute productivity hack regularly into your day in place of checking social media and watch how it positively impacts your to-do lists and helps you feel more proactive.

Chapter 6

Implementation Intentions

Affirmation: I am intentional with my actions to achieve my goals.

Journal Prompt: Think of your habits that cause you the most stress. How could you use implementation intentions to make you feel more in control?

*

One of the easiest and most simple ways of following through and doing what you say you will do is to use implementation intentions.

If you are looking to implement something new in your life, then set solid intentions. An implementation intention is a statement of intent. It is a decision made in advance by yourself declaring **what** your intention is, **when** you will do it and **where**.

In the 2006 review; Implementation Intentions and Goal Achievement: A Meta-Analysis of Effects and Processes by Peter M. Gollwitzer and Pascal Sheeran[1] created the following statements for holding a goal intention and the thought process of implementation intentions:

Holding a goal intention - *"I intend to reach Z!"*

Thought process of implementation intentions - *"If situation Y is encountered, then I will initiate goal-directed behavior X!"*

Putting these statements into action, let's use the example that you want to cycle three times a week [i.e. holding a goal intention - *"I intend to reach Z!"*]

It's a bit too vague for your brain when you don't get specific. Saying you will cycle but not deciding *when* and *where* you will be on your bike could cause you to fail. If you don't at least know when you will cycle, you might not prioritise this activity. That's why using implementations and deciding what, when and where means you have a better success rate of attaining your original goal intention.

Using the above statement, you might say "If it is Monday/Wednesday/Friday evening *[Situation Y]*, then I will *[initiate goal-directed behaviour]* cycle home from work *[Situation X]*".

You have decided **what** you will do (cycle), **when** you will cycle (Mondays, Wednesdays and Fridays) and **where** (on the way home from work).

There have been hundreds of studies into implementation intentions and using them to increase your likely success at achieving a goal. In the above review; Implementation Intentions and Goal Achievement: A Meta-Analysis of Effects and Processes, Peter M. Gollwitzer and Pascal Sheeran analysed 94 studies and the findings from more than 8000 participants who engaged in implementation intention formation on goal achievement. The review noted that there were four key problems en route to goal attainment;

1. Failing to get started
2. Getting derailed
3. Not calling a halt to ineffective behaviour
4. Overextending oneself

Once implementation intentions were used en route to goal attainment, the review findings recorded an effect of *medium to large magnitude*. This was an impressive effect size representing the difference between a goal achievement attained through goal intention vs a goal achievement attained through implementation intentions.

For the last three years I have tried (and failed) to stick to a regular gym routine. When researching this book and learning about implementation intentions, I decided to test them out on sticking to a gym routine. My friend Kelly and I agreed to support one another and we created a plan for the days we would train, the type of exercise we would do on each day, where we would train and what time we would train.

Within the first few weeks of following our plan I said to her "Why does this feel so much easier than any other time I've tried to get fit?" I'd never set a proper implementation intention for the gym before. I hadn't ever made a promise to myself of sticking to set days and times. It had always been a plan to workout three times per week but I rarely scheduled it in on set days making it easy to follow and remember. I'd been using a gym programme that gave me the option of training my upper body or lower body every time I went to the gym. I'd just alternate these as and when I could go to the gym. When Kelly suggested we go to the gym at 6am and follow a routine of upper body on Monday, kettlebells and stretch on Wednesday, legs on Thursday and Bootcamp on Friday - it made it easy. Our decision fatigue of *what* to do and *when* and *where* to do it was taken away. Our need for willpower was reduced as we had a plan. The use of implementation intentions had magnified our success by medium to large effect *(according to the above review)*. I realised why I'd failed to stick to any form of exercise habit and it felt good to finally be in a routine.

Using implementation intentions to plan for when things go wrong

When the COVID-19 pandemic struck and our gym closed, Kelly and I vowed to carry on our exercise routine. I signed up for an online coaching service and created exercise routines to be followed on certain days, just like we had done in the gym. As the above review found, one of the key problems en route to goal attainment is *getting derailed* and implementation intentions can also help you plan for those circumstances out of your control to ensure you stay motivated.

A day before we went into lockdown in the UK, I had an accident when delivering flyers for a volunteer group I had helped to establish. I fell backwards off a neighbour's front step and injured my wrist, knee and ankle. Not wanting to go to hospital amidst the coronavirus outbreak, I didn't get my injuries checked out and had to 'put up or shut up' with the pain. This wasn't part of my plan. While all my friends were sharing sweaty selfies of their home workouts, I literally gave up. My home workouts were impossible as I could not hold even the smallest weights in my hands. I couldn't support my own bodyweight, I even struggled to lower myself to the floor to perform ab crunches and my twisted ankle meant running was off the cards. I literally gave up.

I ended up in a conversation with someone else about implementation intentions around keeping the house clean. I'd got into a smooth routine of implementation intentions like:

- "When I brush my teeth I will clean around the sink."
- "When I put the dogs to bed in the utility room, I will bring clean washing upstairs to put away."
- "When I put my phone on charge downstairs at night, I will clean the coffee machine ready for the next morning."

My friend made an important statement when I was explaining this that was meant as a joke but it taught me something valuable. "So I could use it to say "When the kids have been assholes, I won't drink gin?!"" she asked with a laugh. "Well yes, that could work!" I laughed back.

It made me realise I could use implementation intentions to highlight and therefore stop negative behaviour, or use it to foresee a potential problem and have a positive strategy ready. In the case of my injury I could use implementation intentions to say "When I can't perform my exercise regime at home I can walk for half an hour every day as soon as I get up."

My friend Jaymie Moran at Body Smart Fitness, uses this principle with his clients trying to complete a body transformation. When his clients know they have social events coming up, he gets them to change their habits around food and drink that ensures they stay in a calorie deficit and continue to lose body fat. For example, someone might make a commitment to Jaymie that looks a lot like an implementation intention: "When I am due to eat out, I will check the menu before I go and decide in advance what I am eating that will fit in with my goals." or "When I go out with the girls at the weekend I will drink vodka and diet soda." or "After I have been onion Saturday, I will commit to going for a long walk with the family on Sunday."

Implementation intentions don't just apply to exercise and fitness. I'm writing this now very late at night. I set a goal last week to write for a minimum of 45 minutes a day, every day. As I type about implementation intentions I realise where I have gone wrong. I've been so fixated on my fitness goals and been religious in setting my implementation intentions for exercise, but I haven't done the same with other goals in my life. I have not declared to myself when and where I would type, therefore the day has run away from me and I'm here in bed, with a wireless keyboard typing away to keep my promise to myself! I also think this particular goal intention of writing for 45 minutes every day could be classed as one of the main four reasons people don't achieve their goals; 4) overstretching oneself.

What could I have done instead? Taking away the time commitment of 45 minutes of writing each day and instead replacing it with an implementation intention might work better and feel less overwhelming. Following the formula of creating an implementation intention, I will need to decide when I am writing and where. This needs to be consistent and manageable so I don't overstretch myself and give up on my goal too soon. "When I return from my lunch break every week day, I will open Ulysses and write more on my latest book" could work as an implementation intention in this case.

I can now see that writing after my lunch break will work as it is a time when I can dedicate some consistent effort to the project. When after lunch doesn't work, I need a new implementation intention and this is where a little forward planning with the diary helps. As I sit here typing this chapter (still sitting upright in bed annoyed at myself!) I know that tomorrow is a crazy day for me and I will need to declare in advance when I will fit my daily tasks in so that I can continue my momentum and consistent action. I will be on a train to London tomorrow and returning the day after so my implementation intention is this:

I will write on Thursday at 5pm [WHEN] on the train down to London [WHERE].

I will write on Friday at 7pm [WHEN] I am on the train journey home [WHERE].

Planning in goal actions with implementation intentions

If you are someone who plans out your week or month in advance then setting implementation intentions could be viewed as forward planning. My friend Kate is the most organised person in the world. She works well in advance and has her trusty posh diary by her side at all times. She plans events months in advance including walks, exercise activities and leisure activities. She plans this in first so it becomes a non-negotiable. Anything new coming into her life has to fit in with the things she has already planned. You could set different implementation intentions each week, depending on your diary and your commitments. As long as you have a regular time when you sit down with your schedule, you will have the chance to look at your week or month ahead and plan accordingly.

If you're training for a marathon, you will start your training plan around 16 weeks before your race. Your run distances and training days are outlined in your plan. In order to follow through and complete the plan, you can make sure you plot WHERE you will run and WHEN. These are the missing components to ensure your comfort zone seeking brain doesn't override your weakening resolve to stick to the plan. Joining a sporting club like a marathon training group who are part of a run club can also act as an implementation intention. You commit to a sporting group and the scheduled run times, so it takes that decision fatigue away and you are able to stick to pre-planned training days and times.

If you're trying to study for your exams or write your thesis, you might make a commitment to study [WHAT] in the library [WHERE] on your free study period every Thursday at 1pm [WHEN].

Using the IFTTT (If This Then That) formula

If your goal and intention doesn't fit this formula of I will [intention] when I get to [where] on/at [when] then there is another rule that is slightly different that could help you based on the acronym IFTTT (If This Then That). It explores a different theory of:

If this [scenario A] happens, then that will [trigger scenario B]

For example; If I go to Starbucks [scenario A] then I will not buy cakes [scenario B]. Or another example might be: If it is the 1st of the month [scenario A] I will transfer a percentage of my pay into my savings [scenario B].

The inspiration for the If This Then That (IFTTT) formula comes from the IFTTT free web-based service located at ifttt.com that allows different apps and software to communicate and trigger new action. There are thousands of IFTTT commands and combinations that can be used between services like Gmail, FitBit, your bank, and even smart technology in your home. IFTTT allows you to connect services together so that tasks automatically complete.

It is worth going onto ifttt.com to see if there are handy ways in which you can automate some of your tasks and processes, or even make your life easier. Some great IFTTT examples include:

- Every time you miss a call on your Android phone have it logged as a 'to-do' action in Todoist.
- Track your work hours by location in a Google Sheets spreadsheet.

- Track your mileage and save to a Google Sheets spreadsheet.

- Mute an Android phone when it is time to go to bed or you have a scheduled meeting in your calendar.

- Every time you 'star' an important email set a Google calendar reminder to reply for the next day.

- Get a reminder to drink water every two hours from 8am to 8pm.

- Save money to your Monzo account when you hit your daily Fitbit step goal.

- When Fitbit tracks that you slept less than your goal amount, get a reminder to go to bed earlier that night.

- Get a notification to go for a walk at 8pm if you haven't met your daily step goal.

- Silence all notifications and calls at set times each day.

There's another really good productivity tool that complements implementation intentions called habit stacking. This is the action of linking habits together to take away decision fatigue. As dull as it may be, taking away the need to make decisions when you could systemise your behaviour can be extremely positive.

Now let's look at habit stacking.

Chapter 7

Habit Stacking

Affirmation: My success is a series of positive habits, repeated over time.

Journal Prompt: What are my current automatic daily habits? Good and bad? What new habits would I like to implement in my life?

*

Habits help you stay organised, keep your health in check and keep you productive. If you want to establish a new routine with ease that will see you flying through positive behaviours and stop you putting off certain actions then habit stacking is a must.

This genius little system is so easy and simple to implement. Habit stacking is a way to take advantage of the habits that you currently perform and stack new behaviours onto these existing automatic habits.

You can stack new habits onto any existing habit - whether you deem that habit good or bad. Habit stacking allows you to change your behaviour and create a simple and easy roadmap for your mind to follow every day. It is a powerful memory exercise that will have you forming new habits without it feeling difficult or like a chore.

Habit stacking works very well for establishing a morning and evening routine. Once you are into the swing of using habit stacking at the start and end of your day you can incorporate habit stacking into your work and leisure activities.

How does habit stacking work?

In the same way we outlined the intention implementation formula in the previous chapter, the habit stacking formula works like this;

Before/During/After [CURRENT HABIT], I will [NEW OR NEXT HABIT]

So think of a habit you do daily and make a decision on what you could do preceding, during or after that habit that will help you either get more things achieved, remember important parts of your self care routine or make you more productive.

A simple example might be:

After I have brushed my teeth [CURRENT HABIT] I will wash my face [NEW HABIT]

Or after I have brushed my teeth [CURRENT HABIT] I will floss [NEW HABIT]

Brushing your teeth is a good example of a habit that most people will do daily and without even thinking. Your routine in the morning has featured brushing your teeth since you were an infant and is therefore hardwired in your brain. It is something you do on autopilot and is a good example of the type of ingrained habit you can easily stack new habits on top of.

Your established habit acts as the trigger for the next habit. It's like you are leaving a trail of clues for your mind to follow easily and systematically. At first the road to new habits might feel unnatural to follow, but like a well trodden path you soon walk the route without thinking. Habit stacking takes time and practice so give habit stacking time to embed into your life.

How to create a habit stack

The first part of creating a habit stack is to realise what your current habits are and write them down in full. There will probably be a lot that you do on autopilot every day, so I've provided this list of some common triggers or scenarios where new habits can be stacked or bolted together.

Morning	Afternoon	Evening
wake up	meeting	collect the children
turn off alarm	sit at my desk	get home
get out of bed	make a drink	take off shoes
brush teeth	check email	eat dinner
shower	snack	do laundry
make coffee	make a call	get undressed
get dressed	check my diary	brush teeth
eat breakfast	go to the toilet	change into my nightclothes
walk the dog	finish work	get into bed
drive to work	commute home	turn off the light

Secondly, write a list of habits that you want to start. It is easier to focus on morning and evening routines to begin with unless you work day to day in a role that is already in an established working routine.

Examples of positive habits you might want to introduce into your daily life:

Health	Mindset	Home	Work
stop snoozing the alarm	meditation	do dishes	inbox zero
drink more water	journaling	do laundry	sales calls
walk outside	gratitude	make the bed	plan out day
go to the gym	affirmation	put clothes away	take a lunch

The next step is to look at what you want to achieve with your new habits and cross reference them against your existing automatic habits. Where could you link them together?

Let's say you want to drink more water as your new habit. Look at the morning, afternoon and evening columns at your existing habits and figure out when you could use an existing trigger to drink more water.

After I brush my teeth [CURRENT HABIT] I will drink a large glass of water [NEW HABIT].

Before I go into my morning meeting [CURRENT HABIT] I will pour a large glass of water and take it with me to drink during the meeting [NEW HABIT].

In order to be successful with the above, you might also create another habit stack for the evening that will ensure success the next day; When I go up to bed [CURRENT HABIT] I will take a glass upstairs and leave by the bathroom sink [NEW HABIT]. This means you'll have a glass waiting for you once you've brushed your teeth ready to drink that additional water.

You might create a new habit stack that says; when I get home from work [CURRENT HABIT] I will get a glass of water [NEW HABIT].

You don't need to leave your habit stacks there though. You can use habit stacking to build whole chains of habits that will form a systematic routine.

For example:

Morning Routine

1. When I wake up in the morning I will splash water on my face before I turn off my alarm.
2. After I turn off my alarm I will stretch for 5 minutes.
3. After I have stretched I will journal 3 things I am grateful for.
4. After I have journaled I will change into my gym clothes.
5. After I have changed I will make my morning coffee.
6. While my coffee brews I will drink a glass of water.
7. After I have had my water and coffee I will go to the gym.
8. After the gym I will come home and walk the dog.
9. After I have walked the dog I will take a shower.

Evening Routine

1. When I go up to bed I will take a glass of water with me.
2. After I have put the water in the bathroom I will brush my teeth.
3. While I brush my teeth I will do 50 squats.
4. After my squats/teeth brushing I will wash my face.
5. After washing my face I will get undressed and hang my clothes or put them to be washed.
6. After I have sorted my clothes I will change into my nightclothes.
7. After I have changed I will get my clothes out for tomorrow.
8. After I have laid out my clothes I will get into bed.
9. After I have got into bed I will place my phone on charge, on flight mode and set my alarm.
10. After I have set my alarm I will read for 15 minutes.
11. After I have read I will turn off the light.

These sequences of habit stacks are examples but good ones to demonstrate how a sequence of stacks can make a morning or evening routine flow. Little habits that build like this will add up to really great results. Looking at the above examples as a guide, even small actions like putting your phone on flight mode at night when you go to bed will stop the temptation to scroll for longer than is needed or necessary. You'll probably increase your sleep quantity and quality as you're reading before bed. Setting the alarm becomes the signal to read and reading is a wonderful way to relax and wind down ready for good quality sleep.

How to get consistent with habit stacking

In the beginning you'll need a lot of reminders to help you remember your habit stacks. You might want to write them out like a flow chart or place post-it notes around the areas in which you will carry out your habit stacks. The bathroom mirror and bedside table are two good places to focus on. You might also set alarms in the beginning with reminders of what you should be doing next in your stack.

If you can focus on getting this established into your routine for a couple of weeks, it will become as second nature as brushing your teeth. You will feel like you have more time and you are more productive. Taking care of chores like vacuuming or putting clothes away when you've stacked them onto existing habits means those tasks don't build up as much. They're tackled quickly and easily leaving your home or working environment cleaner and more organised. This then reduces stress in the long run.

Habit stacking 'getting your gym gear on' onto 'turning off your alarm' means you're much more likely to work out. What will consistent working out do for your physique, mental health and energy levels? Quite a lot over a relatively short space of time.

The secret of habit stacking success is to make sure you take the time to do the initial process and write all your habits down. It works so much better seeing your habits all laid out. If you're a spreadsheet nerd you could use excel to outline all your habits and quickly marry them up with new ones. Don't forget to write down the bad ones too! You can use habit stacking to reverse the bad habits. If you are terrible at tidying up after dinner, you can use your evening routine habit stacks to say:

After I have finished eating dinner I will put my plates in the dishwasher > After I have put my plates in the dishwasher I will wipe down all surfaces > After I have wiped down all surfaces I will get the breakfast crockery out for tomorrow.

Before you know it, you haven't just solved the irritating habit of not cleaning up after yourself but you've pre-prepared things for tomorrow saving you precious time and energy in the morning. Habit stacking is an extremely powerful productivity tool and is most definitely worth the initial effort, practice and ongoing consistent action.

Chapter 8

Use the Pomodoro Method

Affirmation: I manage my time effectively. Time is on my side.

Journal Prompt: When I am in a productive state, how long on average can I hold my concentration for? What are the main events, scenarios that break my concentration? How can I reduce these or eradicate them for good?

*

Did your grandma or anyone in the family ever have a simple tomato timer in the kitchen? Usually plastic, red and in the shape of a tomato, these small kitchen timers have numbers around the middle. You twist it and it ticks down from 60 minutes. If you've seen these before, chances are you've used them for timing boiled eggs or a dish in the oven. I love to use one of these tomato timers for a productive way of working. If I had to pick one powerful productivity hack it would be using a mechanical timer to stay focused.

I'm not the only one who loves a ticking timer. A specific technique influenced by a mechanical timer was developed in the late 80s by former student Francesco Cirillo. Taking inspiration from the tomato timer, he created The Pomodoro Technique[1].

Francesco Cirillo found that in his college years he wasn't using his study time well and would get distracted. So he grabbed his tomato shaped kitchen timer and decided to set it for just 10 minutes and focus on his studies - nothing else. He discovered that it was rather difficult to focus on just one thing, but with a bit of time he trained himself and his brain to be focused when using the tomato shaped timer. His 10-minute slots of concentration increased and he found his sweet spot was 25 minutes of focused work on one topic. He developed the Pomodoro Technique which has now been adopted by millions of people looking to focus and knuckle down on their tasks.

What is the Pomodoro Technique?

Whenever you have a massive task ahead that needs to be done (like a final thesis for a student), thinking about the end goal sometimes makes you feel disengaged and hopeless. Breaking down any big goal into smaller tasks is always the way forward to soothe your overwhelmed mind and keep momentum going as you work towards your goal. That's exactly what Francesco Cirillo wanted to do as a student - reduce the overwhelm and break his studies down.

The Pomodoro technique involves breaking down tasks into 25 minute chunks of time. The idea is that you work for 25 focused minutes on ONE TASK and that one task only, and then take a five minute break.

After four consecutive working time blocks, you take a longer break, around 20 or 30 minutes. So your day would look something like this

Pomodoro 1:	10:00	Write blog post
5 min break:	10:25	Get water, toilet, call dad
Pomodoro 2:	10:30	Schedule social media
5 min break:	10:55	Break, water, check email
Pomodoro 3:	11:00	Complete spreadsheet
5 min break:	11:25	Get water, make a call
Pomodoro 4:	11:30	Compile monthly report
30 min break:	11:55	30 min break for lunch

I first discovered the Pomodoro Technique when I was researching my first book, Self Discipline: A How-to Guide to Stop Procrastination. I'd seen a colleague in one of my old jobs use a timer on his phone and break down tasks. I'd dabbled a little in the Pomodoro technique over the years for writing on a deadline but it wasn't until I was writing my first book that I actually put the Pomodoro Technique into regular daily practice.

If you are someone who has to write extensively for a living or you compile reports or work with numbers then this is a brilliant way to focus on your tasks in hand. I'd argue that this is the best method in this whole book of tricks to increase productivity. It is the one technique I come back to every time I need to knuckle down. There's something so simple about setting the timer for 25 minutes and seeing what you can achieve in that time. Going back to the chapter on perfectionism, if you are someone who suffers from thinking your work and tasks have to be perfect then a ticking timer can be a wonderful way to break your perfectionism procrastination and just simply take action without overthinking the outcome.

The way to win Pomodoro

I really love the Pomodoro method and when I am disciplined enough to implement it into my working day it does speed up my productivity, eradicate procrastination and help me achieve more. I started using the Pomodoro Technique in 2015 but it wasn't until 2019 that I really nailed it - and for one good, and inexpensive reason. I had been using a digital Pomodoro timer on my computer desktop or my phone to keep me on track.

While the Pomodoro timer on my phone or desktop did the trick, I was never able to be truly focused for a whole round of four Pomodoros. Something always broke my focus and I realised it was usually due to the action of going to my phone to check the time. Once I picked up my phone, I got distracted by messages and notifications and the focus was broken. I also noticed I tend to stop or pause the Pomodoro timer on my desktop a lot. Because it is digital and easy to do, I would just click pause on the timer. Most of the time I'd end up distracted and not switch it back on. The digital option was too easy to override.

So I went back to basics with a simple gadget - the standard mechanical kitchen timer. Wanting to be true to Francesco Cirillo I shelled out a whopping £10 ($12.50 USD) on a proper traditional red tomato timer like Cirillo would've used. Sadly a little too much heavy handling meant it failed after a couple of weeks and despite trying to take it to bits with a screwdriver, my husband declared it dead.

I noticed in my local bargain shop that they sell these same timers for £1.60 (Around $2) in stylish grey so I stocked up on a couple in case they broke again and they now live pride of place on my desktop. If you follow me on Instagram I will not apologise for my absolute favourite immature pass time when it comes to these timers. Because I love them so much, I buy them a lot for friends or clients. Every time I see a display of mechanical kitchen timers in a store, I can't help myself and I like to twist them all to random times and then walk away. Super childish but so funny watching bemused shoppers' faces as they all go off!

So my childish antics aside, I use this egg timer every day, multiple times a day. It is something so simple yet so effective.

Reasons why I love it over the digital option;

1. It ticks! Like an annoying tick tick tick it is very audible. However, I like that a lot. I like the pace of the ticking and I think it makes me work quicker. I am someone who works in silence with no distractions so the constant beat keeps me feeling focused. If you work in an open plan office, this might not work so great for you - unless you have a coworker who might join in with the Pomodoro Technique?

2. You can't override it. Because it is analogue, you can't 'fast forward' it or pause it. So it keeps ticking and it makes you think "Arghhhh I need to carry on". I think this is how my son broke the tomato one, by trying to 'fast forward' it. It can't be done! If my husband persistently calls when I'm in the middle of a Pomodoro session and I answer, he hears the ticking and knows to not stay on the line too long as I'm trying to focus. I can be a bit abrupt and rude if people call mid-Pomodoro but my family are getting used to it now!

3. The bell is super loud. Once that bell goes the time is up. I like to be in a personal competition with the bell. It makes me feel great when I see what I have achieved ahead of the bell.

4. I use it for cleaning. When I really can't be bothered and I have no motivation for household chores I set the egg timer for 30 or 60 minutes, put on my wireless headphones, listen to a podcast and see what I can achieve in that time. The end bell is loud enough to be heard over the audio in my headphones and again, it's a great way to see what I can achieve in 60 mins or less.

5. It helps with my kid! Seriously! I've started putting the timer on in the morning to speed him up getting dressed and ready for school. As a 9 year old, he has no concept of time but seeing how long is left and hearing the ticking has definitely kicked him into shape in the morning.

6. I've used it to time myself using social media. We all get distracted by the lure of likes and constant scrolling endless updates don't we? I sometimes try to set an egg timer for 20 mins when I'm having my morning coffee. I shouldn't need any longer than 20 mins to comment on posts or check emails or see what's happening with my clients. Any longer than that in the morning is a waste of my life so the egg timer keeps me on track and ensures I get going a lot quicker with my work in the morning. I then use my five minute Pomodoro breaks when working to catch up on notifications.

7. I've used it as a crying/feeling sad timer. This is funny and works. Have you ever been so worked up or so sad that you just want to cry? I'm a big believer in letting out all of your feelings and not keeping them inside. Instead of feeling down for days, set yourself a crying/sad timer. This might be five mins, 10 mins or an hour. Set the timer and ALLOW yourself to feel sad or angry or just have one of those massive snot filled crying sessions. When I set a timer like this, it always ends up in me laughing at myself at the ridiculousness of all this. I quickly start to shift my mood. Not necessarily linked to productivity but if your mood is making you procrastinate then this could be a good little tip!

Grab your own little egg timer from any discount store (get a couple – they do break easily) and see what you can achieve before the buzzer goes off. It's a simple and cheap way to try and achieve more in the time you have available.

Don't forget – try and turn off all notifications, incoming email alerts and all distractions when working this way to ensure maximum productivity.

Other Pomodoro products on the market include;

Focus Booster (www.focusboosterapp.com)
This Pomodoro inspired app is also great for freelancers working with multiple clients. You can time track and tag clients so use this app to report back with time sheets and work reports.

Pomo Done App (www.pomodoneapp.com)
Integrate this clever app into your toolbar for quick click time tracking.

PomoToDo (www.pomotodo.com)
This lets you combine Pomodoro with the Get Things Done (GTD) system. Keep things organised with hashtags and download behaviour reports to audit how you do.

Chapter 9

Create a Tidy Space

Affirmation: My space is a reflection of me. When it is a mess, I am a mess. When it is organised, I am organised. When it is clean I can breathe.

Journal Prompt: What areas of my working space are cluttered and why? What am I holding onto unnecessarily?

*

Hands up if you just can't focus with a messy desk? You are not alone and even those who say they don't mind the chaos of paper strewn desks and disorder, your subconscious could be unknowingly causing your procrastination every time it sees the state of your work space or home.

When our space is a mess, so are we. Even if we don't realise it at the time. While cleaning your desk and workspace can be another form of procrastination or spring cleaning your home can put off other, more pressing tasks, there is a way to factor in a little tidiness to help motivate you into action.

A Harvard Business Review shared valuable research into the effect of an untidy physical environment on our cognition, emotions, behaviour, ability to effectively make decisions and our relationships with others.

Clutter can cause anxiety, stress and overwhelm. Hoarding and the inability to throw items away has direct links with mental health and depression. When we are surrounded by too much stuff we lose focus and it can even affect our eating choices and our sleep quality.

Scientists at Princeton University Neuroscience Institute found that our brains like order. Even if we consciously rebel against organisation, the clutter we can see in our eye line reduces our cognition reserves and significantly affects our ability to focus.

Can you think back to a time when you've done a big spring clean? Maybe you cleared out your closets, drove to the household waste recycling centre and disposed of huge amounts of clutter or you cleaned and spruced your place up from top to bottom. What happens when you finish? You take a step back, take a deep breath, smile and usually let out an audible "Ahhhh".

If it is your desk that is the issue, start by setting a timer. You don't want this decluttering exercise to act as another form of procrastination and putting off the important tasks at hand. Remove everything from your desk and put it on the floor. Clean the top of your desk with anti bacterial spray or polish including your computer keyboard and monitor. Getting it clean and smelling great will help you feel better shortly.

If you have a lot of stray papers and clutter get two cardboard boxes or trash bags. Start to quickly assess the pile on the floor. Mentally mark one box or trash bag as 'trash' and the other 'to sort'. Quickly sift through all papers, books, pens and stationery you collected from your desk and place in either box or bag. If there are items that you will need back on your desk straight away like your mouse, coasters, notebook etc place those back on your freshly cleaned desk.

Once the timer goes off, remove the box and/or bags from your office space and set a note in your diary to tackle those ideally the same day, AFTER you have completed the tasks you've been struggling to get started.

In order to keep on top of your workspace clutter, set regular time aside each week to tidy and organise your desk. It should only take 10 minutes and will ensure your workspace always looks clear and an inviting space to work.

Digital clean

An international survey[1] suggested that paperless office workers lose two hours per week searching out digital documents. While going paperless is still more efficient and with search functions on our computers speeding up the process for locating files, sometimes a digital tidy up can help clear the decks and get you focused.

If you don't already have a good digital filing system, now might be the time to adopt one. Start with your desktop and downloads - the two places that seem to get the most cluttered. What can you delete, rename, move or copy elsewhere? If you set yourself a strict timer for this (I always advise a Pomodoro 25 minute segment of time) you could make great progress that not only helps your digital organisation but getting rid of large and unnecessary files may speed up your computer and therefore speed up your productivity.

Keeping on top of the housework

While the focus of this chapter is the office and workspaces we occupy, we all have homes and we all have household chores we must keep on top of. I am not a naturally tidy person and even though I've been through about four different rounds of Marie Kondo-ing my house I still struggle with keeping on top of the housework - particularly the laundry.

Marie Kondo is a Japanese tidying expert. She has a specific method in her book The Life Changing Magic of Tidying Up[2] and her Netflix TV Show Tidying with Marie Kondo. She has taken people who seem to be suffocating with clutter in their homes and created calm and organised havens for families, couples and singles who had previously been embarrassed by their home environments.

Marie gets you to start to address your clutter category by category, starting with clothes. You are instructed to gather all of your clothing in one space and go through each item, one by one, hold it to your heart and ask "Does this spark joy?" It is a little 'out there' and a little bit nuts but it does work. Depending on your clutter levels, you can expect a whole Marie Kondo process in your home and garage to take a couple of months so it is not for the faint hearted and needs to be completed as a team with the people you live with.

Once you have gone through a decluttering phase, you have to decide where everything goes. If everything in your home has a rightful place it makes it easy to tidy items away and easy to find items you need too. Gathering everything in one place helps a lot. I remember finding six sets of tweezers around my home in various places when I first did this. Now all six live in the same box in the top drawer of the bathroom. Not that we need six, but that's what we accumulated!

The Organised Mum Method[3] is not just for mums. Developed by British blogger Gemma Bray, aka The Organised Mum, Gemma has an app and book to help you break up your household chores into daily focused spaces and tasks. Instead of letting your cleaning and chores build, Gemma motivates her followers to tackle certain rooms and tasks on set days. Monday - Thursday is themed by specific rooms in the home and then every Friday is a focused day for more deep cleaning of different rooms. The idea is if you can dedicate 30 mins per day in this systematic and focused manner then by Friday you will have completed 2.5 hours of cleaning and hopefully won't have to waste your precious weekends dealing with the weekly build up of jobs.

Of course the other thing you could do is hire a housekeeper. I did! I made some adjustments in our outgoings, cut back in certain areas and now I have an absolutely wonderful housekeeper who comes and keeps us organised twice a week. While I still keep on top of the tidying every day, she comes and assists me for those two days to take care of the deep cleaning jobs like mopping, cleaning windows, and deep cleaning the bathrooms. I have had her in my life for a few months now and have noticed a decrease in cleaning procrastination I was definitely guilty of in the past. I am much more productive with a clean office and writing space. I have increased my income by having more time to take more commissioned work and have noticed that I am definitely less stressed in my home environment. Also as a family we have reclaimed our weekends. As the house is cleaned on a Friday our weekends are now spent doing sports or walking or just having fun together - without the worry of a long list of chores. I know not everyone can afford to hire a cleaner but I made some financial sacrifices and made it work for us. It has been one of the best decisions I made for us as a family this year and brings such a sense of peace and happiness.

Chapter 10

Visualise Yourself Productive (Or a Success!)

Affirmation: I am easily achieving all my goals. I have the skills, energy, ambition and talent to succeed.

Journal Prompt: When I look at myself in the future and see myself as a 'success' what am I doing? What am I wearing? How do I look? Where do I live? What have I achieved? What is my legacy?

*

Your brain does not know the difference between what is real and what is imagined[1]. Your brain has no concept of fact or fiction. Which is why if you have found yourself in a past situation you may have sat there in a mild daze, racking your brain to deduce whether something was reality or did you actually dream it?

I remember first learning about this in my mid-twenties. Understanding that your brain doesn't know the difference between reality and visualisation and how it can help you succeed should be taught to all children. It's not too late to learn about it now and use it to your own advantage.

In 2006, working as a radio presenter, I was asked to shadow a local psychologist who ran programmes about positive psychology in schools. Mike Finnigan was his name and he had worked primarily as a sports psychologist for British professional footballers, rugby players, gymnasts and snooker players. He'd taken his work to corporate companies but as a father had been using his work about self belief and changing your mindset on his own young family. This led him to write a book *They Did, You Can*² specifically for children. It told tales of sports men and women using positive psychology to win premier league tournaments, World championships and Olympic medals. When I think back it was actually probably the first self help book I'd ever read. It was excellent. So Mike decided he wanted to take the concepts and exercises from the book and create a programme in schools to help students improve their grades by changing their mindset.

Not wanting to just turn up at the school as a boring psychologist, he took my co-host and I along as the local breakfast show presenters to try and engage the kids. Back then local radio was very popular. It was before the days of Spotify and music streaming so morning radio was a big deal. We were wheeled in as the local Z-list celebrities to endorse the course and hopefully engage the students. It was this encounter that started my love affair with self development and improving your mindset.

We worked with Year 9 students who were aged 13 to 14 years old (for those of you reading in the US that's Grade 8). These students had been chosen to attend these classes because something in their life had changed and their grades were slipping rapidly. Parents getting divorced, bereavement and grief, drugs, crime and getting involved in the wrong crowd had caused these kids to become disengaged in their studies and the teachers wanted an intervention.

Our programme lasted 10 weeks and took the students through all kinds of positive psychology tricks to get them to see the good in every situation and change their thinking.

One of the most powerful lessons from that programme was around visualisation and I still think about those exercises to this day. If you'll allow me to indulge, I'd like to tell you a very short story (you'll see why in a minute).

The story is about to begin and I'd love for you to visualise this story in your mind as you read the words.

It's Christmas morning.

Little Jimmy is lying in bed. He's so excited.

He throws back the covers and tiptoes to the top of the stairs.

Carefully he makes his way down the stairs.

He gets to the living room door.

He reaches for the door handle.

He opens it!

And...

Now take a minute to think back to how this story has been presented in your mind.

When I tell this story in my speeches and schools the chat that follows with the group usually goes like this:

Me: *"How old is Jimmy?"*

Crowd (shouting out): "Five!" "Seven" "Three!"

Me: *"What is Jimmy wearing?"*

Crowd: "Pyjamas"

Me: *"What colour are they?"*

Crowd: "Green!" "Red!" "Blue!"

Me: *"What colour are his bed covers?"*

Crowd: "Spider-Man covers!" "Blue" "Green"

Me: *"How does he get down the stairs?"*

Crowd: "Runs down" "Walks down sideways" "Holds the rail"

Me: *"What does the door handle look like?"*

Crowd: *"Like a handle" "A gold door knob" "it's silver!"*

Me: *"What did he see when he opened the door?"*

Crowd: *"Nothing" "Loads of presents" "Father Christmas!"*

It's funny, this is the first time I've recounted this story in text, rather than verbally and seeing all those answers written down is amusing. They're the answers everyone has given at every talk I have conducted for the last 15 years. These are the same answers from the thousands of people I have done this visualisation exercise with.

At this point in the exercise I say the following:

"OK so let's go back over the story. The facts I've told you are as follows;

little Jimmy is lying in bed

it's Christmas morning

he throws back his bed covers

he goes to the top of the stairs

he gets down the stairs

he opens the living room door

At no point did I tell you how old he was. What if "little" Jimmy is actually 42 and just very small?

Everyone has always said he's wearing pyjamas. Well if he's actually 42 what do you picture he's wearing now?

"Nothing!" "Just his underpants" "A onesie".

The point is I told you the most basic information and you filled in the gaps with the pictures in your mind. You told me colours and ages, textures and methods of movement that I did not tell you. Your brain has created pictures from my words."

I love watching the faces of the teenagers as I do this exercise with them. They're always blown away with how powerful their minds are and it opens up a discussion about using visualisation as a tool to shape future behaviour, reduce anxiety and increase happiness. We go on to talk about the times our brains have created pictures in our mind. How many times have you been told a story and even though you may not have been present, you believe it as truth and you can imagine you were there? That is your brain at work creating pictures in your mind. So if your brain can create pictures in your mind, can it create negative scenarios alongside positive ones? Can you remember a time you were worried about something? Did your mind paint this possible scenario as one that was potentially stressful, upsetting or even life threatening?

Unfortunately we are wired to focus on the negative and as human beings we find it easy to visualise the 'bad'. This is due to our programming that has not evolved as quick as the rest of us. We still respond with the same thought patterns and physiological responses to modern day stress as we did when we were about to be attacked by a sabre tooth tiger as cave people.

So how can you override this visual of doom and gloom and use it to your advantage when trying to stop procrastinating?

Visualise the future you

As you read this book you might be in two schools of thought.

You're either reading this through in full for the first time (or perhaps revisiting it again). Or you're flicking through in a moment of procrastinating stress and looking for a quick answer in this chapter.

Either way, the advice is still the same. Take a moment to think about the one thing that you're putting off and really want to achieve but can't seem to.

Once you have it clear the thing you're procrastinating on, close your eyes. You might want to use some relaxing music and use this as a meditation at the same time. It usually helps with the stress levels.

Close your eyes, take a deep breath and imagine what it will feel like when you have achieved your goal or completed your desired job.

Where are you when you achieve your goal?

How do you feel in your body and your mind?

What emotions are running through you as you achieve your goal?

Who are you with?

What are you wearing?

What else can you see, hear, taste and touch?

Who else is benefitting from your success?

What will be your next step now you have achieved your goal? What will this lead to?

Try and make this visualisation picture as rich as possible and use all your senses to bring it into your mind's eye. The picture in your mind might be you celebrating a sporting win. You might be at your goal weight on your wedding day. You might be handing in your notice. You might be submitting that important report that's going to land you a pay rise. You might be standing in a clean and organised home. You might have sold your home. You might have landed your book deal. Whatever success looks like for you, visualise in as much detail as you can.

Once you have sat with this mental picture for a while, open your eyes and ask yourself what you now need to do to make that feeling and what you just saw a reality. That is going to be your plan of action moving forwards. Go take action!

Chapter 11

Get in the Zone

Affirmation: I am focused, I am energised, I am ready to do my most valuable work.

Journal Prompt: What factors do I need to have in my immediate environment to feel productive? When I am in 'flow' what happens? How can I get myself in the zone for productivity?

*

Have you ever been so focused on a task that it feels like time has stood still? Like no other thoughts have entered your head, nothing is standing in your way, time is an illusion and you're completing things with such ease that it feels like there's no effort at all? You might have heard it being referred to as 'being in the zone' or creative types might call it 'the muse'.

While these phrases are commonplace and have been around for years, it was Mihály Csíkszentmihályi - former head of psychology at the University of Chicago, and author of Flow: The Psychology of Optimal Experience[1] - who named this mental state as 'flow' in 2014.

Being in the state of 'flow' as a concept has gained a lot of popularity since Csíkszentmihályi's research. In our increasingly fast paced distraction deluged digital era, being able to focus and enjoy your state of concentration is what flow is all about. It isn't just doing the work and getting your tasks done, it's doing the work with such peace and enjoyment that it feels like time is standing still and you know this is the work that you were born to do. Creativity and motivation flow out of you with ease.

It doesn't just have to be applied to work and office type work. You can be in 'flow' during a workout or sporting activity, with your partner and social circles, at home cleaning and organising, with your kids or while participating in recreational activities like reading, creative writing, painting, yoga, and music.

Getting into the state of flow requires a level of self awareness about what gets your synapses fired up and ready to put you into this delicious state. We are all different and different factors will affect how 'in the zone' or 'in flow' we are.

We see it in films a lot with sportspeople. Rituals for getting in the zone might get labelled as superstitions but you will have seen footballers and rugby players kiss the ground, or their boots, or have a team chant. We've all seen a team put their hands into a circle, rouse each other up with energetic vocals before reaching up to the sky and shouting their team name for all to hear. What does this do to the brain? They act as stimuli to send the signal that it is time to do the work.

We can also do this in our day to day work - particularly on the tasks we procrastinate on. Get your environmental stimuli right and I'd go as far as saying that these moments where you've trained your brain to get in the zone can become extremely enjoyable, even if you're doing what others might perceive as a dull task.

Abraham Maslow, of Maslow's Hierarchy of Needs[2] fame, called these moments where we are in flow 'extraordinary experiences' and our peak experiences. Maslow stated that in these moments we are at our most fulfilled, unified with ourselves and aware. Maslow even made the bold statement that a state of flow "is the physical manifestation of our true potential".

In order to get into 'flow' you need to focus on the internal and forget the external. Being in flow is about going into yourself and forgetting what anyone else thinks. Yet it isn't something you can directly control. When in flow your brain goes back into default mode, without the worry of negative and destructive thought processes interfering with your relaxed, calm and flow state.

Transient Hypofrontality Theory (THT). Dietrich (2003)[3] suggests that the core components of the flow experience, and other altered states of consciousness, can be explained by reductions in processing by the prefrontal cortex (PFC). Humanistic psychologist, TED speaker and author Scott Barry Kaufman, states that when we are in flow, the 'default mode' of the brain is activated[4]. When we are in flow, the precuneus part of the brain, which is part of the default network, is very active in these moments of creative output. Kaufman argues that this part is the most important for consciousness. During these times, our inner focus on the self, coupled with this 'default' state of the brain is not over complicated by complex thought processes and reasoning. You essentially 'switch off' the part of your brain that controls self-criticism and you are able to perform your tasks with ease or be in that elusive state of 'flow'.

How do you get into flow?

According to Mihály Csíkszentmihályi there are definitive factors associated with getting into flow;

1. You must have clear goals and progress.
2. Your task must provide clear and immediate feedback.
3. You must be at the balance between the perceived challenges of the task at hand and your own perceived skills.

However many researchers have gone on to develop five key factors that must be considered when entering into 'flow';

Self control

It takes willpower and self discipline to firstly get yourself into the state of 'flow'. If you're reading this playing victim to your procrastination then you won't get into this beautiful zone. You have to push past your comfort zone and have self control to get started.

You have to set your own internal standards. You have to decide for yourself and within yourself what you will tolerate and what you won't. Are you someone who is going to get distracted by their phone for the next hour? Or do you have the discipline to move it across the room and out of your reach? What have you been promising yourself that you keep letting yourself down on? Keep those promises to yourself and build inner trust.

Environment

Your immediate environment has the potential to send signals to your brain that now is the time you're getting to work. That might be as simple as turning off distractions, moving your phone, turning off your email alerts or working in a quiet space.

Finding an environment that makes things harder sometimes helps. If a sports person wants to push themselves they may find a harder route, lift bigger weights or swim in a longer pool or outdoor space. In an everyday office, this might be speaking up in meetings or showing off that latest project you created - without fear of judgement from others.

Skills

Because finding that period of 'flow' happens in the middle of something being a challenge and is dependent on a level of talent or skill, you will need experience or a grasp of certain skills in your chosen field. If you're a junior just starting out or maybe you're in a new career with new team members, 'flow' won't come to you straight away. In gaining knowledge we gain confidence and in gaining confidence we get into 'flow'. So practice makes perfect. Practice it over and over starting with the simplest tasks that you're knowledgeable about.

Task

Your task at hand HAS to be something that is important to you. Having a sense of purpose and connecting your work to that is the key to 'flow'. When you are in 'flow' you know what you are doing is probably your destiny and your purpose. When something is so easy and effortless - that is your zone of genius.

You aren't going to find joy in putting in the hours on something you hate or do not care about. So finding those careers or even subtasks and actions within your work that you truly care about is key.

Reward

The reward for being in 'flow' should not come from external sources, but should be intrinsically motivating. While you might give yourself a reward for completing tasks (for example; I will watch that episode of my favourite show with my partner only when I have completed my presentation) this shouldn't be the driving factor.

You should get such intrinsic enjoyment from pushing past your comfort zone and getting into your tasks with ease. While money, rewards and praise can be a positive side effect of being in 'flow', if you're truly in 'flow' they'll never be the overriding motivation and driving force behind getting it done. You'll know when you're in 'flow' when you finish up a task and feel such inner pride and happiness that no other reward truly matters. It is a wonderful feeling and one that when practiced enough enables us to get into 'flow' much easier and quicker.

I'm giggling at myself as I sit and write this chapter. It is 6am on a very cold morning and I haven't slept as much as I'd like. I made a promise I would write daily and report back to my accountability buddy and I knew going to bed last night that the only chance I'd get to do this today would be the early morning. So to get myself in the zone and to provide the right environmental stimuli that tells my brain "Right, it's time to write!" I have the same process and things that are important to me, in front of me. This gets me quickly into a state of flow;

- Journaling
- Incense
- Candle
- Plant
- Oracle cards
- Crystals
- Meditation
- Binaural beats
- No distractions
- Coffee and water

I start my morning with a bit of journaling. Even if it's only for a couple of minutes and even if it's only writing down an affirmation or two it works for me. Today I wrote "I am energised and focused, I love to write. It is a treat and pleasure for me. I love to share what I learn with the world." Corny? Yep! Cheesy? Absolutely! Do I care? No. It works every time for me to remind myself what I am capable of. As 'flow' is a very personal and internal state, I have to do my own cheerleading here.

I light an incense stick that burns next to my desk. This one is called 'energised' and it contains citrus essential oils. I don't particularly like the smell but I like the visual of the smoke as it drifts smoothly past my screen and eye line. The smoke moves in a slow and fluid way and I feel it is very calming. Even though the smell can be a little like fly killer, actually I now associate this smell with focused writing so I find myself enjoying the aroma.

I like to put a plant in front of me when I write. I like to see the green and nature as a direct contrast to my digital, bright computer screen. I also live in a rural area so I can see out the window across the fields if I need a mental break.

A little weird and not for everyone, but before I start to write and another way to get me in the zone is drawing oracle cards. If you're not sure what these are, they're printed cards with different spiritual messages. Some contain just words and affirmations, others contain intricate drawings. Oracle cards have been in existence since the early 19th century and are a spin off of tarot cards. I have no psychic ability but I like the oracle card messages and use them as an affirmation or focus tool. For example, today I have picked one that gives me the word 'will' to focus on today. I like to read the affirmation printed on the card aloud to myself. Today's affirmation is "I have the will to make the changes I need". I stand this card up in a holder next to my desk as a focus piece for the day.

Another little hippy trick of mine is crystals. I have a few in front of me with different meanings. Before I write, I try and take a few deep breaths or if I have time I will squeeze in a meditation. I have a few wand shaped crystals which I like to hold during meditation. I can be a fidget and I find that holding these while I take my deep breaths or do a guided focused meditation helps me quieten the chatter in my brain and get me ready to write.

While I type I will use my over-ear wireless headphones to silence the rest of the world. I use binaural beats as an audio focus tool, usually via the Binaural app on my phone but sometimes I will listen to recommended binaural beat tracks via YouTube.

If I am really trying to focus and have been struggling with my concentration, I will put my phone on a shelf on the other side of the room and disconnect my computer from the wifi so that I can fully immerse myself in writing.

Coffee and water always sit to my right. It feels wrong if I sit to write without either.

Finally, I set my mechanical clicking timer to 25 minutes (my first Pomodoro) and I start to write.

Now I know that sounds like A LOT, but this is something that happened organically for me. It was only when writing this second book that I realised these were the environmental stimuli I had set up for myself to get me in the zone. These all accumulated over a period of a few years but I have now noticed that when I do these things, it is like a switch flips in my brain and I am absolutely 100% ready and usually quite excited to sit down and write.

When I think back to my time working in large open plan offices or my stint working in management for the NHS (National Health Service), I couldn't take candles, incense sticks and plants to place on a temporary desk in an open plan office. I also wouldn't have pulled out the oracle cards there either (for fear the nearby doctors might want to psychologically assess me!). I worked across multiple sites, didn't have my own office and just placed myself on a shared computer or found a power source for my laptop. However, when working in large offices I always had my wireless headphones and binaural beats, used the timer function on my phone to track Pomodoros and used a tracker/journal to keep to time. The Self Journal by Best Self Co always featured on my desk in my office and I'd set out what I wanted to do, then track my intended actions against the actual work produced. This was enough to get me in the zone in my corporate setting and my colleagues soon learned that as soon as my headphones were on and my journal was out that they needed to leave me to focus. It signalled to everyone else that I was busy and unavailable and I always recommend a pair of over-ear headphones for anyone who works in a busy and bustling shared space.

I am not asking you to do the same and I'm certainly not recommending my extensive checklist of things in my environment that put me in 'flow'. You don't need to go out and buy incense and candles and oracle cards. Not at all. I'm encouraging you to be self aware and conscious about what it is in your own immediate working environment that switches you into the zone.

It might be playing your entrance music (as we talk about in the music anchoring chapter), getting a coffee, setting a timer and taking your watch off that gets you in the zone. It might be listening to a particular style of music and using a meeting room away from everyone to do your most focused work. It could even be as simple as taking three deep breaths, stretching, taking a sip of your coffee and you're ready to go. Try to become aware of the little actions you have probably done for years that signal to your brain it is time to focus and get in the zone. Then when you know what they are, put these things into practice and repeat them as often as possible. It makes a massive difference to reducing your stress levels and increasing your productivity when you can line up all the right things that get you out of procrastination and into a state of flow.

Chapter 12

Play to Your Natural Energy Type

Affirmation: I wake up and take full advantage of every day.

Journal Prompt: What do my mornings currently look like? How am I currently using my time in the mornings? What could I do to make my mornings set me up for a great day?

*

Are you a night owl or an early bird? Do you prefer to stay up late and wake later or are you awake as the sun rises and full of energy in the morning? Every one of us operates on the same 24 hour clock but some of us gravitate towards a natural spike in energy earlier in the day and others spike later. Around 40% of the population are classed as early birds, preferring an earlier wake up time and functioning very well in the mornings. The early birds[1] will go to sleep earlier compared to their night owl cousins who maintain high energy levels later into the night. Around 30% of the population are night owls who prefer to fall into slumber later and wake up later. The remaining 30% of the population lie somewhere in between the two types. The morning lark and night owl's natural sleep patterns are known as our chronotypes and are usually governed by our genetics. If your mum or dad were night owls, it is likely you will be too.

Unfortunately, night owls don't have it easy. Modern societal norms have us wake up early to commute and start our jobs and school early. This is not great for a night owl who is naturally predispositioned to wake up later. A night owl's brain remains in a sleep-like state throughout the early morning, even when awake. This can impact our jobs and performance at work. Many chastise night owls for their laziness and believe they should be able to get up earlier and function better. It is not a matter of choice for many night owls, but it is part of their DNA and who they are.

Many books and articles will tell you that the most successful people wake early and follow a set routine and regimen to set them up for a day of success. This is also true and many studies have shown an increase in productivity and happiness by adopting a healthy morning routine. Getting up earlier than you normally would naturally gives you more hours in your day to work on additional projects or participate in events such as running or the gym to help maintain your physique. However, mornings do not work for every single person but every single person can make a conscious effort to make mornings work for them.

Knowing your own natural energy patterns and whether you fit into the night owl or early bird category will help you create the right morning routine for you and your chronotype.

If you are an early bird

If you wake up easily in the early morning then your mornings just became your golden time. You have no excuse why you can't wake up early and create a solid routine of activities to follow each morning that will increase happiness and well-being to help you achieve your goals. Getting out to the gym, walking the dog, running, doing some yoga at home or going swimming are all achievable for you early birds and will help you feel energised and ready for your day ahead.

Hal Elrod's book *The Miracle Morning*[2] has a specific set of activities to follow each morning to increase happiness, well-being and achieve your goals. If you are an early bird you might want to adopt some of these into your morning routine including journaling, meditation and exercise.

You might choose to use your mornings to stay on top of your household chores. If you're the type of person that comes home, eats dinner and is pretty much getting ready for bed then taking care of your household responsibilities in a morning will help you feel like you're able to keep on top of your tasks.

When you're an early bird the world really is your oyster in a morning and you are in a lucky and privileged position to function well at this time of day. Getting more done in the morning will mean it is done and ticked off your list before your day has even begun, leaving you with a winning mindset.

If you're a night owl

Oh dear. It's bad news for us night owls I'm afraid. Even those of us with flexible jobs or shifts might have the luxury of sleeping that little bit longer before work, but the rest of the world doesn't operate on our time. Our partners, our kids and even our pets might not have the same chronotype as we do and the working patterns of our partners or the start time for school for our kids will leave us with no choice but to get up early. I know it's not fair but that is the way it goes. Our task is to work with our natural energy type and do what we can in the time we have available.

Assess if you really are a night owl

Are you really a night owl or are you up late because you're too distracted to go to sleep? Some of us will try with all our might to go to sleep earlier and we just can't seem to do it. If you head into a darkened and comfortable bedroom at a time you would deem as early with no distractions, do you fall asleep? If the answer is yes, you're probably not a true night owl and it's time to assess what is keeping you from sleeping.

Do you go to bed with your phone? Or watch TV? Or read on your tablet? If so, these screens and devices can be causing havoc with your brain waves and keeping you from naturally producing melatonin and that natural need to fall asleep.

Pete's story

> *"I always thought I couldn't get up early in the morning and classed myself as a night owl. From being a kid I'd had a TV in my room and loved computer games. I'd played my Nintendo 64 and Mega Drive for years through to the PlayStation, Xbox and then more recently having my phone with me in bed. I think looking back that I had forgotten how to fall asleep. My bedroom had been a games arcade for over 20 years so I was always up late and found it hard to get up in the mornings. This caused me problems at college and university and then also in my first job.*

When I got married in my early thirties I married an early bird. My wife would be in bed for 9pm and fast asleep after reading her book. She'd moan that my computer games were loud and within the first three months of living together she gave me an ultimatum that the computer games and TV had to go out of the bedroom - or she would be going! I reluctantly gave up my beloved consoles in the bedroom but still found myself taking my phone to bed. I did this for years and would spend a lot of time on social media or news sites for hours after my wife slept.

I started to suffer with depression and found getting to sleep a hard task. I went to see my doctor who was really good in her approach. She didn't want to put me on medication straight away and instead asked me to overhaul my nutrition, incorporate some exercise and look at my sleeping habits to see if it improved my mood. My wife encouraged me to switch my phone off at bedtime and together we created a new sleep routine in the evenings. We kept our bedroom dark and devices were turned off after dinner. Within a week I was falling asleep at the same time as my wife and for the first time in my life was waking up feeling refreshed. I've tried to focus on my sleep since coming to this realisation and I'm genuinely surprised how I feel when I wake up now. In the past I would be awake until around 2am and struggle out of bed at 7:30am to get to work for 8:30am. I was never very productive in work in the morning and so would often work through my lunch or stay late just to finish my work. Once I switched my sleeping routine around I found I was able to go to sleep for 10pm, wake up at 5:45am and be in the gym for 6am. I had more energy and felt better than I've ever felt before. I was also getting a lot more sleep than I had before. I've encouraged my friends and family to get rid of their devices at bedtime too and focus on their evenings to make their mornings better. I feel a lot better in the mornings now and I'm one of those annoying morning people for the first time in my life."

If you've got rid of devices in your bedroom, tried to forge a solid sleep hygiene routine and you're still the type of person to stay up late and wake up late then you need to get creative with your mornings.

If there's one thing I have experienced and know to be true, rushing around in the morning and scrambling to get yourself together to get out the door on time and to work and school on time is one of the most stressful things a night owl does. Actually getting up on time is one of the hardest parts of living as a night owl. Snoozing your alarm 20 times is not going to help you, so what can?

Have an alarm go off in another part of the house - when you're a night owl, sleeping with your phone and alarm next to your face is not going to help you get up. With your brain not functioning efficiently and still being in sleep mode, you will do anything to stop that alarm including turning it off in a semi-sleep riddled haze. If you want to get up on time you have to get up to turn off that alarm. I find charging my phone in hard to reach places shakes my brain into action to turn off the noisy alarm.

Have an accountability buddy when it comes to getting up - who can help you get up on time? I used to have a colleague who called me every morning and would not let me put the phone down until he'd heard me turn on the taps and splash my face with cold water. Sounds crazy? Yes it was! But he did this for many years to help me wake up and get into work on time.

Download an impossible alarm - there's one called Carrot which is truly awful but will make sure you wake up. It demands answers and specific actions to turn off the alarm with pinch movements, pressing moving targets and solving mathematical puzzles in order to stop the alarm. This is not for the faint hearted!

The 15 minute routine for night owls

While our early birds can fit in a few hours of work, a gym session, all the household chores and meditation in the morning, the night owls are lucky if they leave themselves enough time to wash their faces. With the ways to get up sorted, pick your alarm or wake up method of choice and arrange to wake up 15 minutes earlier than you usually do. This is manageable for even the most stubborn late morning riser. Committing to 15 minutes of focused 'you' time in a morning will help you to wake and start your day on the right foot.

Here's my advice for a 15 minute morning routine:

On waking, drink a pint of water. Have a glass ready by the tap for when you wake. The act of drinking cool water will not only help your hydration levels but it will also shock your system into waking up.

Once you have consumed your water, wash your face or get into the shower immediately. There is no better way than water to wake you up. If you can stand a cold shower, even better! This will shock you into getting out of your slumber state.

Once showered, get dry and dressed into your underwear and perform some simple stretches.

This does not need to be a long complicated routine. It is designed to help stimulate blood flow. A yoga sun salutation is a good one to try. You only need to repeat it a couple of times to feel the benefit and it will only take you a couple of minutes.

Get dressed and make yourself a coffee or your breakfast. While you pour your coffee think about three things in your life you're grateful for. Us night owls are renowned for being moody and miserable in the morning as we grumpily go about our day. Putting your mindset into a state of thanks and gratitude has been proven to increase happiness. Put a smile on your face with a little gratitude and enjoy your coffee and breakfast.

To finish your morning routine, play your favourite song as loud as possible. If you've got time to do this at home and dance around - great. If not, play this loud in your headphones as you commute to work or get it on loud in the car. There's no better feeling than playing your all-time favourite upbeat song to ease you into a better energy state for the rest of the day. You will find that when you arrive for work you are less likely to start your day off on the wrong foot of tiredness, grumpiness and procrastination. You will be more energised and ready to start your working day with more enthusiasm.

Chapter 13

Practise Forgiveness

Affirmation: I forgive myself for the decisions and choices I have made in the past. I no longer need to hold onto guilt and shame to punish myself. Every experience is a learning opportunity and a chance to grow into my new future.

Journal Prompt: Where am I being too hard on myself for my past procrastination? How can I forgive myself for my past decisions and choices?

*

Putting off important tasks makes us feel anxious, guilty and even ashamed. The link between shame and procrastination was explored in a 2009 study which sought to prove that self forgiveness could change the way students studying for a midterm exam experienced feelings of shame.

The 2009 study by Wohl, Pychyl and Bennett from Carleton University, Department of Psychology identified that self-forgiveness reduces procrastination by reducing avoidance motivation and increasing approach motivation, manifesting itself in a change in feelings of shame following self-forgiveness for procrastinating[1].

A sample of first-year University students completed measures of procrastination and self-forgiveness immediately before each of two midterm examinations in their introductory psychology course. Results revealed that among students who reported high levels of self-forgiveness for procrastinating on studying for the first examination, procrastination on preparing for the subsequent examination was reduced.

In concluding the study the researchers found that:

> *"Forgiveness allows the individual to move past their maladaptive behavior and focus on the upcoming examination without the burden of past acts to hinder studying. By realizing that procrastination was a transgression against the self and letting go of negative affect associated with the transgression via self-forgiveness, the student is able to constructively approach studying for the next exam."*

The study goes on to say; *"Learning to forgive the self for procrastinating will likely be beneficial by reducing procrastination, but also more generally by promoting feelings of self-worth and more positive mental health."*

Forgiving yourself for past procrastination, whatever it might be that you have delayed, is a stepping stone in the right direction to changing the way you experience feelings of shame around past procrastination. I've interviewed people who feel ashamed they have not saved for their retirement, or put off their studies which will help them excel in their careers. Gently encouraging self-forgiveness and creating a new plan of action to start again helps motivate individuals to increase their feelings of self-worth and self-belief. When a person's self esteem is boosted by self-forgiveness and a reduction of shame, it proves fruitful in increasing self-motivation, drive and productivity.

Forgiveness can come from others too in some circumstances where your past procrastination has affected others. If you promised your wife you would clear your debts so you could get a mortgage but you put it off and now your mortgage application has been denied, you might need forgiveness from her in order to move on. In the main, forgiveness for past procrastination usually starts with yourself and your own inner voice.

Our inner voice can take on many forms and facets. I recently conducted some informal research into how people experience their inner voices and was shocked to learn that not everyone 'hears' their own voice within their heads. Some people see words and images. Some of us are able to have full blown conversations with our conscious minds. Sometimes our inner voice can prove to be a negative and toxic stream of self-conversation. At times, if our inner voice could talk out loud it would be branded as a conniving, horrific and nasty piece of work. Even the happiest and most successful and confident of us fall prey to our own inner critic and negative voice. Yet it is this voice that runs how we think, feel and act.

Overriding this voice is a daily battle when you deal with procrastination. We all inherently want to stay in our comfort zones and getting us out of there only happens when the pain of staying safe and comfortable outweighs the pain of getting our tasks started. Notice I said 'started' and not 'completed', because getting started is always the hardest part.

Forgiving our inner critic

In Debbie Ford's *Dark Side of the Light Chasers*[2] she gets you to become self aware of the inner personality traits that are classed as negative. Once you're aware of these destructive, negative and limiting traits within your personality or subconscious she gets you to give them a name.

For example, when I first discovered this book and accompanying audio programme, I did the work after each chapter. Debbie Ford gets you to personify your personality traits. I ended up with the following characters:

- Angry Agnes
- Indifferent India
- Loud Lorraine
- Procrastinating Polly

I took each of my traits and personified them to view them as a person. I'd visualise what they looked like and imagine them being by my side during key daily moments. For example, Procrastinating Polly was great fun to hang out with but she was always unkempt and ended up being disliked because she let everyone down. I imagined Procrastinating Polly pulling me away from my computer or sitting in front of my face and distracting me when I had to get my head down and work.

A few sessions of visualising Procrastinating Polly and her friends enabled me to move onto the next part of the book which talked about the positives of your negative traits. Procrastinating Polly helped me realise what work I didn't like to do. She made me see the clients I no longer enjoyed working for and the types of tasks I was doing that drained me. I visualised her wanting to protect me from these things. I also visualised moving her out of my way with kindness and promising her I'd be back to chill out once me and Motivated Melissa had spent a working day together. I even remember during one meditation I threw her outside in the cold and said she could come back in when I was finished writing. I explored how Angry Agnes helped me to communicate how I felt. She enabled me to discuss barriers and boundaries. She helped me see what I was passionate about. To counteract the negative personality traits you also think of the positive ones too so Motivated Melissa or Disciplined Donna were direct foes of Polly and I'd sometimes imagine them all battling for my attention with both Donna and Melissa victorious.

This part of the exercise not only deepened the personification of my negative and positive personality traits but it allowed me to build up a story and see that each of these characters were different coping mechanisms. Once I had their good and bad points nailed, their physical features and actions visualised, I was ready for the final part. Now it was time to actively forgive these characters. I forgave Angry Agnes for losing her head at times. I forgave Loud Lorraine for trying to be an attention seeking diva. I forgave Indifferent India for not speaking up and saying what she needed and wanted or fighting for something she believed in. I actually imagined Indifferent India needing a tiny shove from Angry Agnes and Motivated Melissa at times! And then finally Procrastinating Polly I spent the most time on forgiving. I realised she was helping me to find my purpose and calling.

Soon after reading this book and completing the exercise in personifying my personality traits the Disney film *Inside Out* was released. I feel this film really brings this concept to life and if you've got children it's worth a watch. It explores the mind of a teenager called Riley. We get to peek into her cartoon consciousness and find the five key characters; Joy, Sadness, Anger, Fear and Disgust. Each colourful cartoon character represents an aspect of Riley's personality. When Joy doesn't understand Sadness and blocks her out, catastrophe ensues in the mind of Riley thanks to the actions of her personality traits. Anger takes the wheel of her mind with disastrous consequences causing Riley to run away. Joy tries to hold it all together while shutting sadness out only to realise that by blocking Riley from feeling sadness, she stops Riley showing her emotions to others of how she is really feeling and the chance to experience empathy and understanding from others is gone. It is a beautiful film and it helped me with my Debbie Ford *Dark Side of the Light Chasers* exercises to start to make friends with all my traits - good and bad.

Discovering (and forgiving) the many sides of your own personality

If you'd like to do this exercise for yourself in identifying and forgiving the different aspects of your personality traits then follow these instructions:

1. Outline all the aspects of your personality - good and bad. Pay particular attention to the aspects of your personality that keep you in procrastination mode.

2. Give each of these aspects of your personality a name and make them human. What do they look and sound like?

3. Write a two column list of the ways these aspects of your personality both help you and hinder you. Be kind and see things from both perspectives. Yes, you might get angry at times but how does that also help you and prove to be a positive at times?

4. Read the list and see the balance between the two. Forgive the aspects of your personality that have to date kept you stuck.

5. Imagine you making friends with all aspects of your personality characters. It is possible for each personality trait to be a part of you and operate harmoniously. Which personality traits do you need to hang out with more? Which traits need some time on their own?

"The rule of thumb is, you never take action when there is negative emotion within you because it will always be counterproductive. Always talk to yourself until you feel better and then follow the inspired action that comes from that open valve."

— Abraham Hicks.

Chapter 14

List Your Fears

Affirmation: My fears will not stand in the way of my goals.

Journal prompt: What is it I am procrastinating on the most right now? What is the worst that can happen if I do not achieve it? What fears are standing in the way of my success?

*

I was 16 years of age and supposed to be studying for my high school GCSE exams. I was struggling and couldn't seem to get past staring blankly at my revision timetable on the wall. I had it all planned out - weeks and weeks of topics and revision times were outlined. However, the truth was I'd been holed up in my bedroom after school for weeks but hadn't really made any progress. I had some great doodles and plenty of entries into my secret diary but not much actual revision had taken place.

With only a few days to go until my Drama exam and my script gathering dust on my desk, I felt overwhelmed, stressed and helpless. I took out my secret diary, complete with padlock as all teenage girls had at that time, and I started to write. I can't remember exactly how I started the entry but I know I wrote about a life where I failed all my exams, couldn't go to college, couldn't get the grades I needed for drama school and my dreams of being an actress would be shattered. It was a complete catastrophe and completely made up scenario that ended up with me homeless on the streets and living a destitute life.

Of course this was ridiculous and full of unnecessary drama. The truth was if I failed my exam, I would have to re-sit it. I didn't want to do that. The catastrophic future I had envisaged for myself shook me into action and my drama revision became my priority for the next few days. I am pleased to say I gained an A grade, went on to study performing arts at college and although the drama school dreams didn't quite happen, I most definitely saved myself some exam day stress by taking that action and starting to revise.

Over two decades later, I still find myself listing out my fears in some form a few times a week. Even just asking the question "What's the worst that could happen?" is powerful. I've used some form of fear listing when I have had to make really big decisions in my life like choosing whether to put an offer on a house that was a complete wreck and needed completely refurbishing. Or choosing to accept a consultancy role within the NHS (British National Health Service). I've used this exercise when deciding whether to go backpacking for a year and also when my husband and I got engaged quite quickly after meeting and everyone around me said we were rushing into things. It has helped me plan the worst case scenarios for all sorts of huge decisions and made me realise that there's always a way. Marie Forleo's book 'Everything is Figure-Out-Able'[1] rings true in my ears here. There was always a solution and there was always a way out.

I recently had the opportunity to speak at a wonderful event but with only a week to go and a day before the event manager's deadline, my talk wasn't even outlined let alone the slide deck prepared for it. I had other work to finish at the same time and found myself overwhelmed, stressed and procrastinating in spectacular fashion. I knew I could nail this talk. I knew I had the experience, expertise, research and entertainment factor to wow the audience. However, PowerPoint glared back at me. Bare and unloved. Just waiting to be filled with wisdom, knowledge and value for the audience.

I did what I know I always do in these overwhelming moments. I got my trusty journal, Pilot Frixion pen in pink (my stationery of choice), lit a candle, took a few deep breaths and created a sequence of the most powerful fear-inducing questions that would shake me to my core and lead to action:

1. What am I stalling on right now and what is the real reason for my self paralysis?
2. Is any of this based on truth or am I telling myself a story?

3. If I don't take action, what is the worst that can happen?
    - now?
    - in a week?
    - in a month?
    - in a year?
    - in a decade?
4. How does this make me feel?
5. What will it cost me if I don't take action?
    - mentally?
    - physically?
    - spiritually?
    - financially?
6. How will I feel when I take action and/or it is done?
7. What one thing can I do right now in the next 10 minutes to make a start?
8. How long do I estimate it will take me to complete this task?
9. What could potentially stand in my way? How can I make it a priority?
10. Can anyone or anything help me right now?

I answered these questions and realised that I really did want to do the event, but it was my imposter syndrome along with my poor time management that was keeping me stalled. The cost to me of not taking action would impact my self esteem and I was worried I'd lose friends and valuable corporate contacts. There would also be the possibility of a long term financial impact. Of all the things I wrote, the mental and financial cost of not taking action were the things that saddened and excited me at the same time. My mental health is of utmost importance to me but I don't protect it or nurture it when I cause myself untold and unnecessary stress and overwhelm by procrastinating. Realising that a realistic additional income from speaking gigs would accrue a large sum over a decade was hard to ignore. It equally got me fired up into making this first speaking gig on this particular topic absolutely unmissable. I knew that creating an engaging speech would give me the confidence to pursue more paid speaking gigs.

I ran this exercise with a small group of people and collated their answers, reviewing them in the strictest confidence. I then asked each person the question "How do you feel now, after writing that out?"

One person joined an alcohol free programme immediately after answering the questions realising that alcohol and hangovers were causing them to feel shame in some areas of their life and not be as productive, healthy or happy as they could be.

Another person made contact with their tutor of the course they'd been enrolled in and had not completed any of the necessary modules. They secured an extended deadline and we worked together on exercises in self-forgiveness before hatching out a plan to keep them accountable.

One person felt shame around their finances and debts. The questions allowed them to open up for the first time in years instead of being an ostrich about money. They sought out some professional and confidential debt advice and got the expert help they needed. I also shared a few Dave Ramsey YouTube videos and resources. Dave is world famous for helping people pay off their debts early. If finances are your mission with this book, I highly recommend his teachings.

Of the small group who completed the questionnaire, every person was inspired into action after journaling on the questions. It made them realise that their goals were in their hands and they were capable of making a start and making a real difference in their lives.

The questions around what this would cost them in the long term shook them into action but also excited them to behave more positively when working towards their goals. Knowing that a huge financial benefit could happen if you work on your dreams or taking action now could lead to a serious health improvement motivated the group to commit to change. Listing your fears using the 10 questions above helps you audit your present, understand your past and get motivated to change your future. I recommend repeating these questions every couple of months to keep you steering your success ship on the right course.

Chapter 15

Put it in the F*ck-it Bucket and Move on

Affirmation: I do not waste my energy on things I cannot control.

Journal Prompt: "Can I change my current situation? If so, how? If not, can I put it in the F*ck it Bucket?"

*

After researching it, living it, using myself as a guinea pig and writing about all things discipline, productivity and mental health I'm often asked "If there's one piece of advice you could give to someone looking to be more disciplined what would it be?" And the 'F*ck-it Bucket' anecdote and visualisation would be the thing I'd teach to everyone if I could.

Before you can even think about getting disciplined in your actions, building good habits and overcoming procrastination, you have to free up some brain space to even attempt to change.

How much time, energy and stress do we waste on the things we cannot control or change? We get embroiled in dramas about all kinds of topics, people, scenarios and things that really are not in our immediate control. Learning what we can control and learning what we can't control is the first step to taking action. Not only does it immediately reduce stress but it often allows you to step off the cycle of overwhelm, worry and anxiety and approach a plan with a clear head.

Please remember this phrase for absolutely any situation in your life. It is truly transformational. Whenever anything makes you feel sad, worried, stressed, down, anxious or upset ask yourself the following question:

"Can I change it?"

If the answer is "Yes, I can change it, it is within my control" then start to ask more probing questions of yourself to develop a plan of action:

- What am I currently doing that is not helping the situation?
- What could I do more of?
- What could I do less of?
- Who or what could help me?
- When can I do this?
- Why is this important to me?
- What will happen if I don't change it?

If the answer is "No this is completely out of my control" you have two choices:

If the scenario is still really upsetting you or making you stressed ask yourself:

"What could I do right now to make this feel more manageable for myself and/or others?"

If the scenario is a complete waste of your time and energy and is entirely out of your control then you really need to learn to chuck it in the F*ck-it Bucket and move on.

I want to give you a real-world example of this.

In December 2017 my niece Sophia, who was seven years old at the time, came down with a mystery illness. She was hospitalised while doctors ran various tests to try and establish what was wrong. In an absolutely terrifying fortnight poor Sophia was tested, prodded, poked, scanned and screened to try and get to the heart of what was wrong with her. She also suffered with pneumonia at this time too and spending Christmas Day by her bedside while she was attached to all manner of machines was a terrifying experience.

As you can imagine, her parents (my sister and brother-in-law) were absolutely beside themselves with worry. Eventually she was diagnosed with a very rare blood disease which sees a person's own immune system start to attack itself. It is incredibly dangerous and potentially fatal.

This was an awful time for our family. This type of worry and stress has the potential to completely consume a person. My parents were struggling and ended up taking quite a lot of time off to be there for my niece and sister. My youngest sister was at the hospital most evenings. I remember one day being at my desk and trying to write a piece of work. I had started and ended my writing attempts so many times over the previous few days but the consuming worry and wait for news of a diagnosis had me completely paralysed.

My friend Kerri first introduced me to the F*ck-it Bucket concept and she was by my side at this time listening to my worries and stress. She asked me a really important question. "In this whole situation, what can you put in the F*ck-it Bucket?"

I went for a walk to clear my head. Trying to find any positive in the situation, I wrote down a list of everything that was good in this present moment. I realised that Sophia was in one of the world's best children's hospitals. She had a private room. She was under the care of the UK's leading rheumatologists. While I may not be able to control her disease and I may not be able to beg the Universe to take it away from her, I still had the ability to be grateful that her diagnosis had been caught early and she'd survived. I could still be grateful that she was being cared for by exceptional clinicians. I could still be grateful that our whole family was rallying round to take care of her younger brother, my nephew, and we were all there for each other.

While it would be wrong and dismissive to put this whole scenario in the F*ck-it Bucket, I realised I could put my worry and anxiety in there for sure. I was doing myself and my own family no favours by being paralysed with fear. My work was suffering, my home life felt wrong and I needed something to focus on.

So I asked myself the question above "What can I do to make this situation more manageable for myself or others?"

I started to think of the ways I could offer my help. I could be there on the phone for my sister and brother in law. I could visit when visitor numbers would allow. I could bring supplies and snacks. I could take care of my nephew. I could call my parents and younger sister to check they were all doing OK.

I also asked my sister what I could do to help. "Can you come and visit and just make us laugh?" she asked. I had tears in my eyes as I answered "Of course". I headed over to the hospital that day and kept the situation light and fun, trying to find joy and light in the dark moments. I drove home from the hospital feeling lighter and brighter. I felt like I'd used my energy in a way that benefitted and helped myself and others. It definitely made the situation more manageable.

Create your own bucket

It's your choice. Your own F*ck-it Bucket can live figuratively in your head or you could actually buy a bucket, write 'f*ck-it' on the side of it and when shame, sadness, stress, guilt, negativity, heartache and all those things you sometimes just cannot control crop up in life - chuck them all in and think "f*ck it!". You could choose to write down your worries or the things you can't control on pieces of paper and toss them into your bucket. At the end of the month, look back on all the stuff that could've tied you in knots.

I choose to keep mine in my head but my friends and I do encourage one another to use the f*ck-it bucket when scenarios crop up that cause too much unnecessary stress.

That awful mother on the school playground? *F*ck-it Bucket.*

Online grocery delivery got cancelled so you have to eat toast for dinner? *F*ck-it Bucket.*

Jim the office asshole got the promotion over you? *F*ck-it Bucket.*

Got a parking ticket? *F*ck-it Bucket.*

The F*ck-it Bucket might be a better way for you to practise that all important, scientifically proven self-forgiveness for reducing future procrastination. If the idea of being loving and kind to yourself when offering forgiveness doesn't appeal then a magical bucket where all your f*cks go might be a better option.

The F*ck-it Bucket will allow you a vessel to visualise what is done, is done. As Elsa from Frozen famously reminds us - the past is in the past as she lets go of all her shit. You just can't change the past so stop wasting any more time and brain space stressing about it.

The PG-rated Chuck-it Bucket

If you need a PG friendly version of the F*ck-it Bucket, name it the Chuck-it Bucket. Same concept and principle applies. Take all that stuff you have no control over, release your attachment to it, don't get involved in the energy or the drama of it and just chuck it in the bucket!

Chapter 16

Write Down Your Wins

Affirmation: I am always in harmony with the energy of winning.

Journal Prompt: What have I achieved so far this year that I would deem as a 'win'?

*

Are you a fan of writing down a long 'to-do' list of everything you need to get done? The concept is simple - write down all the things you have to do and tick them off as you do them. Easy. Yet it isn't easy is it? If it was, we'd all be flying through our to-do lists every single day.

What happens when the to-do list overwhelms you and leaves you wide eyed and whimpering into your notebook rather than chomping at the bit to take action? The antidote is the anti to do list! For this chapter, we're going to completely forget about what needs to be done in the future and we're going to look to the past for clarification that this too will pass and we can emerge victorious over procrastination.

Research conducted by Harvard Business Review[1] studied the best ways to fuel innovation among teams of ordinary scientists, marketers, programmers and other knowledge workers. The research found that innovative people are driven by the power of progress and celebrating wins *as they happen*.

The research saw knowledge workers keep in-depth diaries of their working day and researchers noticed a phenomenon they labelled the 'progress principle'. According to the diaries, of all the things that boosted the workers' knowledge, motivation and mood during a working day, the single biggest factor that had the most impact was making progress in meaningful work. The more progress workers made and the frequency of days where progression was noted, the more people were likely to be creative, productive and therefore innovative in the long term. It was determined by the research that everyday wins, even small ones, made workers feel different in how they feel and perform.

In a nutshell the research is common sense: do the work, make progress, celebrate the win = feel happier and more productive. The part of this equation that is the most difficult to master is stopping to celebrate or even notice the win. Sometimes you can feel so overwhelmed with all you have to do in a day that you complete one thing and then quickly move on to the next without stopping to appreciate what you have just achieved.

This is one of the reasons I really love working with the Pomodoro Technique (as outlined in chapter 8). When you force yourself to focus on one task and one task only, when you complete it and you note it down, it is there in black and white for you to see what you have achieved. Rather than getting pulled in all directions and feeling like you don't make any tangible progress, focusing on one task allows you to systematically work at it, complete it and then feel a sense of achievement once it's done and you're working on your next Pomodoro.

Another example of the power of celebrating achievement and wins was evident in the marketing campaign for Febreeze. When Febreeze was launched as the antidote to all nasty household smells, the marketing team for Proctor and Gamble wanted to make a song and dance about the power of the product. Through beta testing the early formulas of the household air freshener and scent removal spray, the company was able to note that the product didn't just work, but it worked better than anything else out there. They gave a bottle of the formula to a woman who worked as a park ranger and frequently caught skunks as part of her job. Every day she would come home and her ranger clothing would be overpowering with the stench of the skunks. It was in her hair, car, home and was affecting her dating life. She loved the product so much that she broke down in tears about how it has changed her life and allowed her to socialise more without the fear of the skunk smell.

The marketing for Febreeze in the early days was all about masking odours; dog and cat smells, sports equipment, sneakers. The adverts depicted us spraying all the stinky things around us. Febreeze wasn't selling nearly as well as it should for something so powerful that could mask the most overpowering stenches.

So researchers began rolling out product testing to a control group who were observed on video or in person using the product. Soon, through repetition of watching the habits and behaviours of the control group, researchers discovered one common behaviour that could be the answer to their marketing problem. At the end of the cleaning session, once the control group had vacuumed and mopped the floors, sprayed the cushions, dusted the surfaces and tidied items away, they tended to then stand still, look around, take a deep breath, and breathe out a satisfied smile. A "Ta dah!" moment to show that everything was done and they were happy. Each one was celebrating their hard work with a quick scan of their achievements and a fleeting moment celebrating their win. This moment became the new focus for marketing Febreeze. The new campaign depicted home owners finishing their cleaning, quickly spraying Febreeze, taking a deep satisfying breath (at the smell of the Febreeze) and then smiling. This one relatable cue and reward put Febreeze on the retail map because it matched our typical human behaviour.

Writing down your wins daily is a wonderful exercise. It also forms part of a gratitude list for some, or I do have a friend who writes a 'glad list' every evening on social media outlining all the things that happened in the day that they were glad about. Their business and personal wins are documented daily and it's such a great thing to read and be inspired by. I know she gets a lot from writing this down every day.

This book is all about overcoming procrastination so I don't want to overwhelm you by adding more things into the mix if you're currently stuck and feeling held back by your own stalling behaviour. If you're not yet ready to add this into the mix, consider writing down your wins regularly in the future when you've improved your productivity.

If you've flicked to this chapter for a quick prescriptive process for overcoming procrastination then consider the following exercise that brings your wins of the past into your consciousness.

Write down your wins

Sometimes in these moments of procrastination a little reminder of the success you have achieved in the past works well to help you see a clear picture of your capabilities on paper. Focusing on the past has the power to take you from dithering to driving into the future with positive action.

Taking the time to write down your wins from yesterday, last week, last month, last year or even your lifetime (if you're really feeling in a dark hole and you need to crawl out of it) will show you that you've been a winner before, and you can be a winner again. Maybe you could cast your mind back to a time just like this. When was the last time you were procrastinating as bad as this? What did you do to get out of it? What were the circumstances and outcomes? Did you get it sorted in the end? If so, how did you do it?

Write down all the times you have really procrastinated but in the end took action and made progress.

Maybe it was that time in January after a heavy Christmas that you finally decided enough was enough, laced up your trainers and went to a gym class.

Maybe you could throw back to that moment when your house was a tip and you were embarrassed at the thought of having family to stay. You sat stressing about it for ages but eventually you rose up, got started and got it done, then emerged proud at the look and smell of your home.

Maybe you could recall a time when you really needed to get that report in for work and put it off for such a long time. You were so stressed about it but in the end you made the time, took the action and completed the important task.

It doesn't matter how big or small these actions were in the past, the point is to list as many as you can. I'd suggest setting a timer for this exercise because if you are in the grips of motionless momentum, you don't want to use this exercise as another form of putting off your tasks.

Step 1

- Get a piece of paper and make two columns
- Set a timer for 10-15 minutes max
- In the first left hand column, write down every battle you've had with procrastination. Just keep writing and try not to overthink it. What things have you stalled in the past and caused yourself additional stress? Write as many things as possible in your time limit

Step 2

- When your timer stops, have a look at your list
- Ask yourself what things stand out? What tasks have you procrastinated on in the past? Are there any patterns?
- Circle 3 key moments from the list that stand out to you. Circle 3 wins that you're particularly proud of. Maybe you feel that relief again just reading them that you were able to overcome the delay and achieve your goal. Pick moments that feel good

Step 3

- Set your timer again for 5 minutes max
- In the right hand column, next to the three key moments you have outlined, write down what your trigger was for finally taking action? How did you feel at that moment? What was it that took you out of inaction and spurred you to make a start? How did you achieve this goal?

Step 4

- Look at your answers. Take a moment to appreciate how you have got through this in the past. How did you overcome these moments that previously threatened to derail your progress?
- What can you take from this exercise that will inspire you into action right now? How have you done it in the past? What was your battle plan? How did you execute it and get yourself out of No Man's Land?

Step 5

- Remembering back to that time when you took action and won, how can you channel how you felt in that memory to get started right now?

The Ta-Dah list (rather than the To-Do list)

So once you complete the exercise above, you'll be fully aware of your previous wins. You will have noticed the patterns of behaviour that spurred you into action and hopefully it will have cemented in your mind that you are adept at getting yourself unstuck! Always remember - you've done it before and you can do it again.

Now as you get started on your tasks today, instead of writing a to-do list of everything you need to get done, why not start to collate a ta-dah list? A what? Yes, a ta-dah list. (Imagine someone quite showbiz with splayed hands exclaiming "ta dah!" when they've done a good job.) This is a celebratory list where you keep track of everything you've achieved in your day, rather than looking at a long to-do list and feeling disgruntled and annoyed that there's so much to do.

A friend of mine keeps a page a day diary by her bedside and every evening writes about the best thing that happened that day or the things she achieved that she's proud of or happy about. If she ever needs an instant pick-me-up she goes back over her little book of wins and feels fantastic.

Chapter 17

Create a Lightbulb List

Affirmation: My mind is for creating ideas, not storing them.

Journal Prompt: What niggly things have been on my mind this month that I need to address or action?

*

We've covered a to-do list and a retrospective ta-dah list but what about those thoughts and niggly things that fly into our minds just as we are trying to take action, or mid-project?

You have probably experienced this yourself. You're in the middle of a run or a really important report and your mind just keeps wandering to something you've been meaning to do for ages. You end up having an internal conversation of commands:

"Call grandma."

"Book the dentist appointment."

"Send flowers to my cousin."

"Renew the car insurance."

Many of these things are completely mundane and really frustrating to think about when you're in the middle of something else. You can often get so distracted that this is the thing you are thinking about right now and you can't take any further action until it is addressed. If you do this often enough and multiple times while trying to remain productive you'll find you don't get much done. Getting distracted, even for a few minutes, adds up when it happens time and time again.

Alternatively you might spend a lot of mental energy batting these thoughts away and never actually action them. A fortnight later you're driving around in an uninsured vehicle, your toothache has become unbearable, grandma hasn't heard from you and your cousin's birthday was missed. Those things you didn't get around to end up causing you even more stress in the long run.

How do you get over these incoming thought streams and create a system for dealing with them effectively?

I like to keep what I call a Lightbulb List. Those moments little lightbulbs go off in my head, I now choose to honour them, listen to them, list them and then turn off that light in my mind promptly. I use the Pomodoro Technique when it comes to focused work so in my longer Pomodoro breaks, if I am not preparing food or out walking I will address those things that have floated into my mind and see if there are any quick wins I can get by solving them straight away. This is the important bit when it comes to a Lightbulb List as continued action really helps your mind feel accomplished. If your list is too long and hasn't been tackled in days then it will be yet another overwhelming list that will stress you out. Taking rapid and continued action gets your mind into a state of feeling accomplished. Do this often enough and you'll find the wandering thoughts become less frequent. Rather than spending a few days thinking "Renew the car insurance…renew the car insurance" as you're trying to focus, you'll have reviewed your Lightbulb List, taken action and that recurring thought won't be popping into your head multiple times a day and distracting you.

How to store a Lightbulb List

If you're a pen and paper type person, a simple notebook is effective for passing thoughts. Just make sure you have it easily to hand as you're working so you can add your lightbulb moments into it without too much interruption.

Thin post-it notes on your desk also work for this. I use thin post-it notes, write actions down on them and stick it on my desk or computer screen. It helps you to keep on track with your work tasks but it also works in terms of lightbulb moments. Add them to a thin post-it and once actioned, rip it off the desk and throw it away.

You could use apps like Evernote, your notes on your phone, Todoist, Wunderlist, Asana, Trello and a whole host of other apps on the market to keep lightbulb moments. Create a specific list and add to it every time one of those fleeting thoughts grazes your consciousness. I use both Asana and Trello in my daily work as a copywriter and I use Asana in great depth for keeping on top of my book writing and all the actions needed. I don't use either for my Lightbulb List though as I find it a distraction looking at the other tasks on my list of things that need completing.

Also if these lightbulb moments come to me at a time when I am not in 'work mode' I find myself naturally resisting Asana or Trello. I am quite disciplined in separating work from home life these days and delving back into Asana on a Saturday never works. I find I have this natural resistance to add anything to it if it is an evening or weekend. If I'm at the farm shop and the thought of "Buy more pens" enters my head as I go to scratch off my shopping list and the pen runs out, it isn't Asana where I turn to record that.

I found the thing that works best for me is WhatsApp. I use WhatsApp multiple times a day. It is how I connect with my husband, family, friends and clients. I use it round the clock on both my phone and my computer so for thoughts that enter my head around the clock it is the perfect place for me. I created a group called 'Lightbulb List' and added my husband into it. Then I deleted him. Much to his confused bemusement. "What's this group you've added me into and then took me out of?" he messaged with curiosity. Adding someone into a WhatsApp group then removing them leaves only you in the group and allows you to essentially send notes to yourself. As I use the desktop version of WhatsApp on my computer, I can also add thoughts as I'm working quite easily. I then pin the group to the top of my WhatsApp view meaning I always have it to hand and it is the first thing I see when I log into the app.

I have to admit that this system works the best for me of all the apps and systems I have tried, but it does have a downside. If I am trying to be focused and I'm writing to a deadline, or I am writing a chapter of my latest book or I am lying in bed awake (I don't have my phone by my side overnight) then I don't have WhatsApp close by. In this case I will shout at Siri to remind me to add these thoughts to the Lightbulb List at a time I know I will have my phone. I charge my Apple Watch by my bed so it picks up my voice as I shout "Hey Siri. Remind me at 6am tomorrow to add 'book Blake's check up' to the lightbulb list". The next morning when that reminder pops up it displays on my phone. I open up WhatsApp and add that to the Lightbulb List which is saved and pinned to the top of my view.

My husband and son are Android lovers, not Apple users so they do something similar with Google. My husband is known as 'Google Shaun' in our circles as he has been shouting "OK Google" into his phone for years to get the answers to all his burning questions, set reminders and get directions. My son is only nine but uses his Google Home device for things like "OK Google. Remind me at 8am on Friday to take my swimming kit to school". Yes, it makes me one proud mama to witness him taking advantage of technology and keeping a Lightbulb List in his own way.

Using voice commands to keep a Lightbulb List comes in very handy when you're driving. It isn't possible to write into a notebook when you're driving but shouting at Siri, Google or an in-car system that is voice activated works really well. Some in-car systems let you send voice activated WhatsApp messages which is great if that's your system. If you are out running then voice commands can keep your lightbulb moments in a list. Equally even activities like swimming can be paused while you shout orders at your smart watch. It has never been easier to capture your thoughts using technology. It is getting into the habit of it that takes a little time.

Reviewing the Lightbulb List

It is really important to regularly review your Lightbulb List. If you're not in a routine with it, like in the midst of a Pomodoro Technique inspired working day, then these little thoughts can build and build.

Depending on the frequency of you adding tasks into your list, I recommend having a fleeting glance every morning or evening to see if there is anything you can action right away. Every week have a more in depth review of the list and if things are no longer relevant, get rid of them. I tend to review my list on a Sunday. Sometimes these items I have added are proper work tasks that might take collaboration with others. I might migrate them over to Asana or Trello if I need to get feedback from other business partners. I'll assign a person and deadline to them so they form part of my daily workflow and tasks.

Find a system that works for you

As with absolutely everything in our lives, you get to find a system that works for you.

If you're reading this chapter right now and you're in the midst of procrastinating then create your first Lightbulb List in a format you know you will check regularly. It could be a post it note on your desk, a notebook by your bed, a list on your iPhone, a lost app, Facebook Messenger, text, email, Instagram DM to your business partner, Snapchat to your best friend, a note on the fridge or a note to your PA or VA to help keep the list for you. Use a platform that you check the most often, that way it will be at the forefront of your mind. Clear it little and often and you will soon feel like you're achieving more and more. You'll free up valuable brain space and stop the distraction and interruption of tasks that haven't been tackled and keep weighing on your mind.

Chapter 18

Pick Your Winning Music Track

*

Affirmation: I behave like the winner that I am.

Journal Prompt: What music track gets me in the mood for action? What song energises me?

Have you ever seen the beginning of a boxing match? What do the fighters do? They come into the ring to a specific predetermined piece of music that means something to them. It's the music that gets them fired up and ready in their winning mentality.

Do you have a must-listen track that instantly gets you fired up?

We all have music we hold an emotional connection to that impacts our brain waves and can change our mood. Music has that great power to change our conscious emotive state. There will be songs in your life that instantly take you back to a moment in time, a memory or a person.

Do you have a song from a time in your life that acted as a pick-me-up? Maybe you played it driving to a crappy job you hated, or you'd play it as you got ready for a big night out? Maybe you played in a sporting team at one time and you had a signature song that was synonymous with your sporting buddies? Maybe there's a song from a night out celebrating your exams or that long, hot summer before you started college?

If you don't already have a piece of music think of a song that is going to be YOUR anti procrastination track. It's going to be your song that you come into the ring with and knock out procrastination in one punch.

Don't pick something drab and dreary. Don't pick something that is going to make you cry or think of someone you have lost.

What is that one song that you're guaranteed to dance to when it comes on in a club or a bar or at your best friend's wedding?

My winning song or piece of music is:

So the concept of this book is for you to get out of procrastination and into a productive state. That is why this chapter on music anchoring is in two parts. The part above is about picking that one song that is going to ignite a fire in your belly, change your state and get you primed for productivity.

Before we move on in this chapter, I want you to go and play that song you have outlined above. Your winning song needs practice. Just like Pavlov's dogs started to produce saliva on the sound of a bell before being fed, we need to prime your mindset for productivity and it takes a little practice. Play the song. As loud as you can. Ideally if you have headphones even better (so you don't disturb others). If you don't know the lyrics by heart, get them up on your phone or the computer. If you can, sing along. Loud. Put all of your energy and passion into it. Doesn't matter if you're tone deaf and can't sing a note. Rouse that noise inside of you and sing it loud. Listen to it all the way until the end.

Right, now play it again a second time. This time don't worry about the lyrics if you don't know them, hum along if you have to.

Stand up.

Press play. Again, loud as possible.

Now, start to move. With as much energy as you can muster, move. Dance. Jump. Run. Twist. Just move! Get your synapses firing as you move with as much speed and energy as you can. If you know the words sing too - loud!

Dance and sing all the way through until the end of the track.

Sit down.

Get ready to play your track a third and final time. This should NOT be a chore for you. This is your most favourite high energy track in the whole wide world and you could listen to it over and over and over again for days and hours.

Before hitting play, take a deep breath and check how you feel. Your heart should be pumping. Your cheeks may be a little flushed. You might need to get some water! Feel this energy, this action, this movement. It was all bottled up inside of you and now you've unleashed it. Capture that energy, keep it with you.

This time play the track again a little lower in volume and close your eyes. As you listen to the beat and the lyrics, imagine yourself full of boundless energy every time you hear this track. Imagine the dullest, most awful task that you hate most. The one you ALWAYS procrastinate on. Imagine you are about to attempt to do that task, but first you are going to listen to your winning song. Imagine yourself in the scenario of that task. Visualise yourself dancing energetically and singing loud just before you start that task. Imagine yourself protecting this energy from this drab task. It will not take away from your fun and your favourite song. Your favourite song is a privilege to dance and sing along to. Imagine yourself using this song to get in the zone every time anything in your life feels difficult or you're avoiding and resisting it. This is YOUR song. This is you in your own ring of productivity, knocking out your own previous resistance and laziness, perfectionism and procrastination with one swift punch to each.

When the song ends slowly open your eyes and take a deep breath. Smile. You've just started the process to programme your brain for success.

Important: OK so some of you reading this are going to freak out at that. "What if someone sees or hears me?" "This is stupid. I'm not doing that." You might feel embarrassed or like it is pointless but trust me, give it a try. Even if you're just listening to your winning song in your headphones and visualising yourself dancing and singing and full of energy. It all helps put you in the right winning state and mentality.

You could use this track on your way to work in the car, on your way to the gym, on your running playlist or even just play it at your desk through your headphones when you're about to start that important piece of work.

Music for continued productivity

You are not going to listen to your winning song on repeat for your 8 hour working day (it will soon turn into a hellish song rather than winning song if you listen to it too much). So what can you listen to for increased productivity?

Firstly that depends on you personally. Even though I am a radio broadcaster there is absolutely no way I can listen to the radio in my work day-to-day as a writer. It is too distracting and I can't focus. I also can't listen to generic music in the office, the gym or at home. You will pretty much find me wandering around or working at a desk with wireless headphones in at all times. Confession - sometimes they're not even switched on! Sometimes I just have the noise cancelling function on.

One thing I do find incredibly helpful and very weird is binaural beats, but these are so powerful I've dedicated a whole chapter to them as I'd really like you to give them a try.

Classical music

You may have heard of the 'Mozart Effect' which relates to a study by researchers Gordon Shaw, Frances Rauscher and Katherine Ky[1]. The researchers tested out the effect of Mozart on three groups of students. The first group listened to a Mozart selection. The second group listened to a relaxation tape. The third group listened to nothing and sat in silence. At the end of the listening period, all 36 students were subject to a blanket test. The group that had listened to Mozart averaged an 8-9 point IQ increase compared to the other two groups.

This study came under fire years later with some scientists stating that the enjoyment of the music had increased the mood of the students, their productivity and therefore their results. So the test was repeated on rats who were played Mozart in the womb and for 60 days after birth. A second group played minimalist music by composer Philip Glass and the third group played nothing - just silence like the original experiment with the students.

At the end of the listening period, the rats were tested on their ability to negotiate their way out of a maze. The rats who had listened to Mozart completed the maze much quicker and with fewer errors than the other two groups. Testing the rats proved that musical enjoyment and appreciation wasn't a factor in the test.

The music played was Mozart's sonata for two pianos in D, K448. As I type this I am currently listening to it and I am not normally someone who can bear any kind of music while writing. I am struggling to focus, but I will test it again as per the experiment above. I will listen to the track again and then write immediately afterwards.

In a study published in the journal Deutsches Aerzteblatt International in 2016, researchers compared the music of Mozart and Strauss with that of ABBA on issues related to heart health[2]. The results from the experiment showed that people who listened to classical music by Mozart and Strauss had markedly lower blood pressure and their heart rates had decreased. Sadly ABBA's music did not have the same effect.

Many historical classical musicians created music that has stood the test of time and continues to be used for pleasure and relaxation. I remember my own first encounter with classical music was during visits to the dentist. My dentist always had classical music on while you sat in the chair. My sister and I were always considered strange compared to our classmates when we did not share the same fear of visiting the dentist. Maybe this was because it was always a very relaxed encounter thanks to classical music? I always enjoyed our visits and enjoyed the music very much.

Another time I saw classical music in action was in a problematic high school. I was hired to deliver positive life coaching workshops to students aged 14 who had started to fall behind with their studies. The school was a difficult school in a deprived area with a history of violence and terrible exam results. A new head teacher introduced classical music during all recreational breaks during the school day and had seen a dramatic decrease in violent altercations and an increase in mood. Some teachers had started to adopt a classical music playlist in the classroom during focused work. We did the same during week 2 of our workshops and noticed a positive difference in concentration levels of our students.

Nature sounds

You may have heard of whale music or the sound of rainfall to relax but could it also work for productivity?

The Journal of the Acoustical Society of America conducted psychophysical data and sound field analysis on subjects who listened to 'natural' sounds or 'nature noise'[3]. The data suggested that listening to waves on the beach, the sound of birds singing, rainfall, jungle sounds and whale music could enhance cognitive functioning and increase your concentration.

There are multiple nature inspired playlists from streaming services like Spotify to create the right ambient setting inspired by nature.

Your favourite tunes on a playlist

While this might not be the right soundtrack for focused and complex work, if you're trying to stop procrastinating on repetitive work tasks, household chores, running or training in the gym then you might want something more high impact and upbeat to spur you on.

With most digital streaming services these days it is really easy to put together your own specific feel good playlists. Gone are the days of taping your favourite radio show on cassette (and pausing when the advertisements would come on!). You can also even create a playlist of your favourite music on YouTube.

You can split playlists however you like. Maybe a pounding heavy metal guitar inspired powerful playlist for weight lifting, the best of the 90s for cleaning and an easy listening chill out vibe for the office. Putting playlists together is really fun and can really make a difference to your mood, your focus levels and your energy.

*As I come to the end of this chapter I've just finished listening to Mozart's K448 in full and actually it was rather pleasant. The other Mozart track cited in other studies is K488 Piano Concerto No 23. I've just pressed play on it and it's much more sombre and slow and actually making me feel depressed! Isn't music amazing the way it does that?

Chapter 19

Binaural Beats

Affirmation: I am focused and achieving my goals.

Journal Prompt: What sounds help me the most when I am trying to focus?

*

If you are struggling to focus and get complex tasks completed then consider trying to listen to binaural beats.

A binaural beat is the illusion of two different noises set at different hertz or wave patterns to create a whirring or buzzing sound. It is an auditory illusion perceived by our brains when two different waveforms, each with a frequency lower than 1500Hz, but less than a 40Hz difference between the two waveforms, are played at the same time.

For example if one tone of 530Hz is played in the left ear and one tone of 520Hz is played in the right ear, the brain will perceive the auditory illusion as a binaural beat with the perceived pitch being the difference between the two of 10Hz, otherwise known as binaural beats in the alpha range.

In order for binaural beats to create the auditory illusion of a buzzing or whirring sound, each waveform needs to be played to the listener dichotically - one sound through each ear. Which is why in order to get the benefit from binaural beats you will need to listen to them through headphones.

Binaural beat ranges:

- Gamma (39-50Hz) good for problem solving and complex complicated work
- Beta (13-39Hz) good for general activity and focus on any task that doesn't require your audible attention
- Alpha (7-13Hz) good for relaxation and dreaming
- Theta (0-4Hz) good for deep sleep

Our brains process these differing and somewhat clashing waveforms by sending auditory signals and electrical impulses from each ear along neural pathways into the brain.

Binaural beats are popular in productivity circles for people looking to reduce stress, alleviate anxiety, increase a person's focus and concentration, improve motivation, increase confidence and assist deeper meditative states.

However, a 2015 study by Becher et al took all the available research on binaural beats to test whether they do have a positive impact on mood, reducing anxiety levels, improving memory, creativity, attention, mood and vigilance[1]. Researchers working on the study concluded that there are only single studies to support the findings and many lack consistency. The only consistent finding was that several studies reported binaural beat stimulation reduces anxiety levels. How anxiety is reduced, however, is still not yet understood.

I have been listening to binaural beats for over five years in my work and they are my best tool for staying focused and in my own flow and bubble. If they have been proven to reduce anxiety then this makes sense to me. I use binaural beats when I am writing for myself or speed writing (copywriting) for clients. I often enter into these periods in an anxious state. If I am working for clients I am against the clock and am always under pressure to write at speed. If I am writing for myself I often feel guilty about it which causes anxiety. I feel I should be spending my time working for clients or being a good wife or mum. Putting on the headphones and listening to the binaural beats always acts as a little way to truly hide and focus. So while these beats may not have been proven to actively change my brain waves, I definitely work quicker, with less anxiety. I write with more accuracy and in a state of relaxation with these sounds in my brain.

Listening to binaural beats is not for the faint hearted and does take some getting used to. If you are someone who really struggles with persistent and continuous noises you might get no benefit from these sounds and instead just find yourself frustrated and annoyed. There are some binaural beat tracks on YouTube that directly tackle this by mixing up the Hz of the beats in one track so that it is not a continuous and monotonous sound.

If you are going to try utilising binaural beats to focus and take you out of procrastination, you do need to be careful that you don't listen to them for extended periods as they can cause headaches. You will know how it sounds to you and whether it causes any discomfort so test it out and see how you go. If you feel any form of dull ache, stop listening.

You will also notice that once you take your headphones off, if anyone speaks to you or you speak yourself, the speech will sound distorted and like a Dalek from Doctor Who! It always freaks me out how this noise affects the ear's ability to process sound for a minute after listening to the binaural beats.

You can download binaural beat videos from YouTube, access binaural beat tracks from your favourite music streaming service or download specific binaural beat apps. I have one simply called 'Binaural' from the app store that allows me to select an appropriate binaural beat frequency for my desired activity. There is also an app called 'Relax Melodies' that allows you to mix your chosen binaural beats with guided meditations, music and other nature sounds whether you're looking to focus, relax, meditate or sleep.

Chapter 20

Have a Power Nap

Affirmation: I know when to rest. It is good for my well-being.

Journal Prompt: How do I feel if I take a short nap in the daytime? Does it energise me or make me feel more tired?

*

Taking yourself off for a nap might seem like counterintuitive advice for someone who procrastinates. Have you ever had so much to do that you've actually just taken yourself off to bed in the middle of the day? (Guilty!) However scientists suggest that getting sleep for a certain amount of time is the difference between waking up refreshed and raring to go compared to waking and feeling like you've been run over by a bus.

There are three different modes of sleep;

Monophonic sleep - a period of sleep within 24 hours (this is what the majority of us do).

Biphasic sleep - the practice of sleeping over two periods in 24 hours.

Polyphasic sleep - refers to someone who sleeps multiple times in a 24 hour period, usually more than twice.

Segmented sleep or divided sleep may refer to the practising of biphasic or polyphasic sleep but it can also refer to interrupted sleep, where a person has one or several shorter periods of being awake (think new parents dealing with the sleep deprivation challenges of a newborn or the poor insomniac).

However many people, thanks to the research of sleep on the function of our brains, believe that taking a power nap in the day (or practising structured biphasic or polyphasic sleep) can have a positive impact on our mood, stress levels and productivity.

Massive companies have adopted daytime dozing as part and parcel of the working day and office culture. The super offices of Ben & Jerry's, Zappos, Uber and Google all contain dedicated sleep spaces in their headquarters. Employees are able to take themselves off to sleep pods during the working day. It is a more modern spin on the traditional lunch break but employees often report a boost in creativity, positivity and productivity after 40 winks in the sleep spaces.

In The Journal of Sleep Research, 2009 review Kimberly A. Cote, PhD, a psychology professor at Brock University in Ontario, states that even in well rested people, naps can improve performance in areas such as reaction time, logical reasoning and symbol recognition. Cote also stated that power naps could be good for the mood[1].

But how long should we power nap for? During sleep, adults cycle through a series of sleep stages, with a single cycle lasting about 90 minutes. Dr Sara C Mednick is associate professor of Psychology at the University of California, Irvine and author of the book, *Take a Nap! Change your Life*[2]. She specialises in research around sleep and cognition. "In a 90-minute nap, you can get the same learning benefits as an eight-hour sleep period," Mednick says. "And actually, the nap is having an additive benefit on top of a good night of sleep."

If you can spare an hour and a half, which is a lot longer than the average lunch period for most workers, this is a good length for a nap that will cover all the different sleep stages. Sleeping halfway in this period between 40 and 60 minutes could have an adverse effect and leave you feeling groggy and worse than before your nap started. In the middle of a sleep cycle you will switch from REM sleep to deep sleep which is much harder to wake from. So if you can't spare that full cycle of 90 delicious minutes for your nap, the recommended amount of sleep for a power nap to help boost cognitive function is around the 20 minute mark. You must also take into consideration the time it takes you to fall asleep, otherwise known as your latency. If you take 20 minutes to even fall asleep then taking another 20 minutes on top of that is going to seriously cut into your lunch hour.

If you work from home a nap in the day can be dangerous. Sleeping in the bed you usually get your nightly rest in tells your brain it's bedtime and the tendency to want to sleep for longer can overcome you. This is the complete opposite of what you want when you're looking for a solution to stop procrastinating on a task!

Personally, I can't do short naps unless I am laying on a hard floor and I am following a guided sleep meditation. If I attempt a short 20 minute power nap in my bed you can guarantee I will still be there hours later and my night time sleep will be affected. I've tried the 90 minute cycle too and it just doesn't work for me, I wake up even more tired. I have also noticed since wearing my Oura ring and tracking my sleep that if I have a sleep in the daytime this really impedes my night time sleep quality. Asking other people on the Oura ring support groups yields similar experiences - naps are not always for everyone. On the flip side, Ben, my accountability buddy who helps me focus on writing my books, takes regular naps in his work day. Ben works from co-working spaces and finds the bean bags and chill out zones the perfect place to shut his eyes for 20 minutes and feel refreshed. He's able to come back to his work and tasks with more zeal.

You could try taking a power nap in your car at lunchtime and try it out. Have an alarm set to make sure you wake up and give it a try to see if you emerge from your car slumber feeling more energised.

If you'd like to try some power nap guided meditations then the Insight Timer app has lots of these in differing durations depending on the time you have available to sleep. I also like to use Andrew Johnson's hypnotherapy apps[3]. His soothing Scottish voice and timed hypnotherapy works in harmony with our natural sleep cycles and he gently raises his voice to wake you from your naps.

Other apps that are worth testing are Pzizz which states it can get you into REM sleep quickly and get you out of it before you fall into that deeper sleep phase. Loved and publicly reviewed by JK Rowling, Pzizz audio programmes include voice narrations based on clinical sleep interventions. Things like diaphragmatic and heart rate variability breathing, grounding, mindfulness meditation, guided imagery, somatic awareness, progressive muscle relaxation, autogenic training, hypnosis and more. It's an impressive roster of sleep aids to help you feel more creative and get you into a problem solving mode on waking.

Another more basic app for the iphone is the Power Nap app. It uses relaxing sleep sounds and sets timers to control your wake up time from your naps. Power Nap is not nearly as intuitive and well researched as Pzizz but it does boast not having a heart-attack inducing alarm when the time is up. Great for some but worth bearing in mind if you're someone who struggles to rouse from an afternoon slumber session. We don't want you getting fired now do we?

Chapter 21

Have a Coffee Nap

Affirmation: I can accomplish great things today with coffee in my hand

Journal Prompt: Sit with a cup of coffee in your hands. Try and clear your mind of all other thoughts and take note of the temperature of the cup, the smell of the coffee, the taste and aftertaste. When the cup is half full, close your eyes and take a deep breath. Notice the first thing that comes to your mind. Write about that moment in your journal and what came up for you.

*

So we've already talked in the book about the productivity boosting powers of a nap in the middle of your procrastination pressure, but what about a coffee nap?

If you hate coffee you might have to move on from this chapter, although they say that tea has as much caffeine as coffee and some energy and soft drinks are laden with caffeine. While it is not something I'd want to actively encourage you to try, if those are drinks that feature in your daily life anyway, feel free to experiment with alternative caffeine sources.

Drinking coffee before a nap might sound like complete madness but there are studies to show the benefits of a nap directly after caffeine[1].

In your brain, an inhibitory neurotransmitter called adenosine acts as a central nervous system depressant. In normal conditions, adenosine promotes sleep. After we wake, the levels of adenosine in the brain rise each hour.

If you are tired it may be that your adenosine levels are elevated. Once you fall asleep, these levels begin to decrease again.

When you drink caffeine, it competes with adenosine for receptors in your brain. It effectively prevents your brain from receiving adenosine and you feel less tired and drowsy. Which is exactly why caffeine can help reduce tiredness levels.

So, if you want to really boost your energy levels in a double hit, drinking caffeine and then sleeping will cause your body to naturally decrease adenosine and the caffeine won't have as much adenosine to compete with for the receptors in your brain. So coffee on its own will increase the availability of receptors for caffeine in the brain but the decreased adenosine will also provide an energy boost too. Put the two together and there's double the energy you may have felt just drinking coffee or having a nap.

Won't the caffeine stop me from napping?

Not necessarily. It takes around 15-20 minutes for caffeine to work at reaching the receptors in your brain. So if you drink your coffee and get your head down straight away for a nap for 15-20 minutes, by the time you awake from your nap your caffeine should be ready to give you that energy boost.

If you are napping for 30 minutes or more, you may fall into a slow-wave or deep sleep. If you wake up in the middle of slow wave sleep it can actually make you feel more drowsy and disoriented. So limiting your coffee naps to less than 30 minutes can avoid this. If you're also going to take a nap in the middle of your working day you want to know that you'll be able to wake up OK and also be feeling refreshed, rejuvenated and ready to tackle your next tasks. Use a daytime nap app or loud alarm or timer to ensure you stick to napping for under 30 minutes.

The exact time of the day when you decide to take a coffee nap is also important to note. A study of 12 adults found that those who had 400mg of caffeine, the same as four standard cups of coffee between 0 and 6 hours before bed all had disrupted sleep.

You may have felt this yourself when drinking coffee or caffeinated drinks. If you have them too late in the day they can really impact your ability to fall asleep in the first place and sometimes to stay asleep. You may already have a 'coffee cut off point' in your day (mine is 3pm!).

When considering the benefits of taking a coffee nap, the amount of caffeine you consume before your nap also plays a part. Most research agrees that 200mg of caffeine, around two standard cups of coffee, is the amount of caffeine you need to feel alert after waking.

Black coffee is also best. Adding milk, sugars and sweeteners could impair the caffeine's ability to reach the receptors in the brain. Elevating blood sugar levels may cause a crash soon after which can induce further drowsiness and cause an energy slump.

So taking all of the research into account, the best advice seems to be no more than 200mg of caffeine, consumed immediately before napping for 15-20 minutes and nap more than six hours before your eventual evening bedtime.

Please note that excessive caffeine intake is not for everyone. Some people experience anxiety, palpitations, restlessness, headaches and other health issues. It does disrupt sleep for many people so you might think that taking a midday coffee nap will help boost your short term energy levels, but at what cost for your overall sleep quality?

Health experts agree that around a maximum of 400mg of caffeine a day - the same as around four standard cups of coffee - is safe for most people.

If you do experience anxiety, heart issues, impaired kidney function, poor sleep or headaches please do consult your physician before considering coffee naps as a solution to daytime productivity levels.

Chapter 22

The Power of Accountability

Affirmation: I am accountable for my words and actions.

Journal Prompt: Where do I need a bit of accountability in my life? Where would it help me to have someone cast their eyes over my goals and actions and keep me accountable to achieve them?

*

Whether you like accountability or not, it works. There's science to prove it too.

When it comes to exercise, a 2013 study published by researchers at the University of South Carolina found that sharing your weight loss goals and journey on Twitter had a direct impact on the amount of weight lost[1]. Researchers deemed 10 Twitter posts about the subject's weight loss progress equalled 0.5% weight loss. Putting the goal and intention out there in the public domain makes you behave differently. In Gretchen Rubin's book, *Better Than Before*[2], she writes "Accountability is a powerful factor in habit formation, and a ubiquitous feature in our lives. If we believe that someone's watching, we behave differently." There is even a study that suggests watching *yourself* could help. Psychologist Roy F. Baumeister and science writer John Tierney chronicled studies into accountability in their book *Willpower*[3]. One study proved that even having the presence of a mirror, so people could watch themselves, made people more likely to work harder and resist temptation.

Then there's the phenomenon of Pearson's Law which states: "When performance is measured, performance improves. When performance is measured and reported back, the rate of improvement accelerates." We actually perform better at work when we are accountable to someone because it gives us a sense of purpose, guidelines and goals to aim for. While Pearson's Law is regularly quoted in strategic performance within businesses this same principle can be used for almost anything that requires discipline from sporting endeavours to weight loss. Having someone else to report back to and be accountable to dramatically improves performance.

One of my clients is an online fitness, nutrition and mindset coaching company. Called Body Smart Fitness, Jaymie and his team of coaches help bring out the best in people. The reason why they are so successful with their client results is the different levels of accountability they have in place. They encourage clients to make small, realistic and positive changes to build new habits and change the identity they want for themselves. They are not face-to-face trainers and do all of their coaching via video call and WhatsApp. However their clients do maintain honesty and transparency in their reporting processes. There is a weekly check-in process which includes weights and measurements along with happiness, sleep, hydration and stress ratings. They encourage clients to send videos of themselves performing resistance training movements with weights so they can keep them accountable with their technique and form. Then they might request that a client struggling with their food takes a picture of every meal and snack they eat. They also provide personal 1:1 coaching calls and group coaching calls to all collectively share experiences and learning. It also adds a little competitive element when they bring different clients together to communicate each week. This extensive approach to accountability works in two ways:

1. The client is less likely to 'cheat' and cut corners knowing that they have a coach watching over their progress.
2. They want to do well and they want praise from their coach so they adhere to the plan and instructions for the reward of praise each week. They are also rewarded with results.

This accountability relationship continues until the client has surpassed their goal and made their new habits an effortless part of their daily routine. If a client leaves their coaching relationship too early, before they've embedded their new actions into their daily life, they tend to struggle without accountability.

A coach in the situation above acts like an accountability partner. You might also instruct an accountability buddy in a friend, family member, colleague or peer to be your new gym partner, running mate or mentor at work. Accountability partnerships are very powerful when they're done well. A good accountability partner will be consistent with communication, have the confidence to challenge you and also act as a supportive and encouraging cheer leader as you work towards your goals. The American Society of Training and Development (ASTD) did a study on accountability and found that publicly committing your goals to someone gives you at least a 65% chance of completing them[4]. However, having a specific accountability partner increases your chance of success to 95%.

The only reason you are reading this book is because of Ben, my accountability partner. We have been helping one another with our goals since January 2016. It started out as a WhatsApp conversation between the two of us before migrating over to a carefully labelled Trello board. In the past year we've gone to higher levels of productivity and use Asana - a work management and collaboration platform to keep on top of our tasks. Ben is super efficient with Asana and has created a foolproof system where we assign tasks and due dates to one another while leaving each other clear instructions on the tasks that need to be completed. Every morning when I have my morning coffee I use the Asana app on the phone, go into my tasks for the day and my inbox to see what needs to be achieved and completed. It took us a while to get used to this style of working but we are now like a finely tuned machine and it flows effortlessly. I am attempting to write a book in a month later this year and will use Asana to track my daily word count and report back to Ben how I have done with my writing each day. Without the notifications from Asana and Ben's eagle eyes watching over everything I do I know this goal of publishing books would possibly remain a dream that is never fully put into action. Having accountability most certainly helps us both keep momentum on our projects and continue to check off daily actions that move us towards our ultimate goals.

It doesn't matter whether those goals are business or personal, when you decide on a goal but don't take any specific strategic and consistent action, the goal will not be brought to fruition. Fortunately, a study by the Dominican University of California has created what they believe to be the magic formula of achieving goals and guess what? Accountability features prominently within this formula alongside commitment and writing down one's goals[5]. Let's take a look at it more closely.

Dr Gail Matthews led the study as a direct response to the discovery that the Yale (or sometimes cited as Harvard Business School) study of goals was a fake urban myth. Dr Matthews with the help of Steven Kraus, a social psychologist from Harvard, debunked the myth in which the 3% of the graduating Yale class that had specific written goals went on to earn 10 times more than that of the remaining 97% of the group with no clear goals. Despite proving that no such study existed, this 3% figure was discussed in many business circles prompting Dr Matthews to study how commitment to goals and accountability would help goal success.

A group of 267 participants were recruited from businesses, organisations and business networking groups with only 149 participants completing the study. Participants were aged from 23 to 72, with just under three quarters of the participants female. Participants resided in the United States, Belgium, England, India, Australia and Japan and included a variety of entrepreneurs, healthcare professionals, artists, bankers, managers and educators.

Participants were put into different control groups with some asked to write their goals, and others just to think about them. Of all the groups of participants, the group that committed to the following reported the most goal success:

1. Commit to action - the first stage of the process was to write a goal and then commit to achieving it. The group members were guided through a thorough thought process via a survey which encouraged them to set their goals and decide in advance the necessary action commitments.

2. Be accountable to their peers - the group members had to outline their concrete actions and plans to an accountability partner. They needed to send this commitment to their peer and that peer would check up regularly on their progress.

3. Provide regular updates on their progress - in addition to the accountability partner checking on their commitment and consistent action, the students had to update their accountability partner on their progress on a weekly basis to keep them focused on their progress.

The outcome of this study showed that those who sent weekly progress reports to their accountability partner achieved significantly more than those who had unwritten goals, just wrote their goals, formulated action commitments or sent those action commitments to a friend. There was also a positive correlation between public commitment and goal achievement; those who made their goals public noticed an increase in success.

Get some accountability right now

If you're stuck in the midst of procrastination right now and need a way out of it or you have a goal in mind that has been something you have had your heart set on for a while then it's time to get accountable.

Firstly, write down your goal. Even if you have done this many times before, this is a new page on your next chapter so write down your goal and what you want to achieve. In the short term it might be filing your taxes, cleaning the house or even making a start on that weight loss regime. Whatever it is, write it down and get specific with the end goal. Don't make it too vague.

Now write down as many things as you can think of that you will need to do between now and achieving your goal. Again, if it is something as short term as cleaning the house, why not outline the jobs that need to be completed. Don't take too long on this because writing lists can be a form of procrastination too!

Now looking at your lists and your actions, how can you become accountable and get those done? Who or what can help you? If it's the state of your kitchen could you send a 'before' pic to your best friend and ask them to hold you accountable to send a pic in an hour once you have conquered the mess? If it is filing your taxes, could you create it on a spreadsheet online such as a Google sheet that your accountancy advisor or trusted friend or spouse can also see you working on. Set an agreed time limit you will work on the taxes and report back to your accountability buddy. If you want to lose weight could you commit to that gym class you have had your eye on? Who could go with you and also keep you accountable to attend regularly?

There are many ways to stay accountable. If you don't have a trusted friend, spouse, sibling or parent who will dedicate the time needed to hold you accountable, what about getting professional help? Coaches help keep people accountable in many areas of their lives from business to health. Could you hire a coach or join a group programme online to help you stay accountable?

Could you post publicly about your journey? I have a friend who has two big boxes in his kitchen. Each box is filled with polythene bags of sand. He's weighed them out and each bag is 1lb in weight. One box represents the weight he wants to lose, the other box represents the weight he has lost. When he weighs himself weekly, he moves the appropriate number of sandbags across to the success box. It provides a great visual for him to stay on track and he posts about it on Facebook. I love seeing his progress like this visually and I like the idea he has it in his kitchen. Another friend has a wooden-cut-out that sits on her counter top. There are spaces for 50 £1 coins to be placed in there. For every 1lb of weight she loses, she places a £1 coin in the wooden slot as a reminder of all she has achieved so far. Again, I only know about this because she posts pictures of it on social media.

I am part of a running club and many of our club members are currently in training for the London Marathon. They regularly post updates of their latest runs including their times, distance and heart rates as an image from Strava or Runkeeper. They enjoy the feedback and praise they get from others when they make themselves accountable in this way and we enjoy following their progress.

A friend of mine entered his first bodybuilding show a few years ago. I helped him vlog the process and we created a weekly entertaining vlog about what he'd been eating, how he'd been training and the different aspects that led up to competition day. Not only did this generate interest from his friends, family and clients but the encouragement along the way and knowing he would be on camera getting filmed every week spurred him on to work harder. He ended up going on to win that competition and said the weekly progress report via the vlog kept him focused.

If you are struggling to stay focused in your day to day role and you're reading this book because you want to improve your performance at work then which trusted colleague can help you? Or do you know anyone in your sector who possibly works for another non-competitive business who you could learn from? Could you engage with others via LinkedIn groups or Facebook groups who understand your role and who can share best practice ideas? Or do you simply need a better way of reporting your work so that you don't slide off into procrastination and then end up feeling not good enough in your role? Even those at the top with no direct boss or business owners need someone to bounce ideas off and stay accountable to. Does someone else you know run a business? Could you create your own mastermind style meet-ups with a group of friends in person or online to share your business ideas, challenges and goals?

There are many ways to stay accountable and many of them require a certain degree of bravery, vulnerability and visibility. The science and the data do not lie though. If you want to get your stuff done and take action then accountability is one of the very best tools in your anti-procrastination kit.

Chapter 23

The Accountability Mirror

Affirmation: I am proud of the person who looks back at me when I look in the mirror.

Journal Prompt: Write down a list of everything that you judge yourself for. Next to each point you make, write 'I am enough' and write a short reason why you are enough against each one.

*

I have been listening to David Goggins talk about his use of the accountability mirror in his audio version of his best selling book *Can't Hurt Me*[1]. David Goggins is a former Navy SEAL and ultra marathon athlete. He has raised millions for charity with his sporting endeavours, is the world record holder for the most number of pull ups in 24 hours and is described by some as the 'hardest man on the planet'. The audiobook version of *Can't Hurt Me* is narrated by his ghost writer Adam, but David is also there for the recording of the book. The two men regularly stop to discuss the content in the chapters and elaborate on David's life story making it feel like a podcast and audiobook in one. I highly recommend it.

Throughout the pre-written book chapters and the additional bonus discussion, David references his use of his accountability mirror throughout his life. It started when he decided to change his identity in school from 'straight out of the Hood' cool kid to preppy student ready to learn. He made a decision one night looking in his bathroom mirror that things had to change. If he had any chance of getting out of his situation and poor upbringing and making something of his life he needed to study and he had a dream of getting into the military. So the low slung pants were replaced with chinos and his "I'm too cool to learn" attitude was transformed into a dedicated young man who improved his exam scores and got his place at college.

Every night David would stare at his reflection in the mirror and ask if he'd done the best he could that day. Had he given it his all? Got out of his comfort zone? This interesting yet powerful concept of having a silent conversation with his reflection followed him through his first job while in the Air Force and then his dramatic 106lbs weight loss in three months to enable him to try to be a Navy SEAL. His daily self discussion with the accountability mirror saw him go through the gruelling Navy SEAL 'Hell Week' (he is the only person to have gone through three separate Hell Week processes!), combat in Afghanistan, treacherous training with both The Rangers and Delta Force.

In the book and bonus content in the audiobook he talks of times he shouted at his reflection in that mirror but on the whole this process was a calm, cool and collected exercise designed to reveal his truth.

Marisa Peer is a hypnotherapy specialist and British therapist who is widely known for her 'I am Enough' mirror concept[2]. The difference between Peer's approach to Goggins is that she gets you to write on all your mirrors "I am enough" and repeat it back to yourself every time you look in the mirror. This is a contradiction to Goggins' approach which was always one of "I am NOT enough - I always have more to give". (I warned you this book would feature contradictions.) You have to decide which tactic is right for you when it comes to procrastination and achieving your goals.

I'd encourage you to try both ways. The hardcore approach and the self love softer approach. Which one is the most effective? Which one moves you into action? Feeling enough already or feeling like you aren't and you could achieve so much more?

I've regularly written about my own battles with self discipline around food. The side effect of years of binge eating and food addiction was a 50+lb weight gain and a complete change in body shape. For years I'd tried every self discipline trick in the book to shift the weight. I used the accountability mirror concept for this in a few different ways. First I tried the 'I am enough' approach. It made me emotional every time I would stand there in my underwear and try to say the words out loud. I would find myself going on to say things to myself in my head like "I am not my size." "I am not my weight." "I am not fat, I have fat." "I can change this. It is in my power to do so."

Undoing years of self loathing and hating my body was a long process. I naturally gravitated from saying "I am enough" to learning acceptance at my body image in the mirror. I caught sight of my own facial reaction to my reflection one day. It was a split second conscious realisation at the self hate and self loathing that had become my new normal every time I looked in the mirror. I knew something had to change. I knew this negativity was so damaging and was keeping me stuck. Just standing there and hating what I saw rarely spurred me on to eat better to head to the gym.

So after seeing that facial expression flash across my face I knew things had to change. I made a decision there and then that EVERY time I looked in the mirror I had to be completely conscious in my reactions. I had to smile, soften my scowl and look at my body with love and gratitude. I decided initially to try this for 30 days. It was honestly the hardest thing I've ever done. My instant reaction was to turn away or cry. "How did I let it get to this?" was a phrase that constantly entered my consciousness. I also made a pact and a promise to myself that I'd stop pulling at my skin in the mirror. I realised I'd spent years grabbing at my waist or my soft tummy, bottom, thighs and boobs with such violence. I'd never in a million years let anyone else grab me in such a harsh and painful way - so why was I doing it to myself? I changed every belly grab, muffin top pinch, boob uplift and bum flatten to actions that were consciously soft and loving. Again, this was so unnatural and difficult. I was actively practising self love. I'd guess if I were David Goggins this would not be his military approach but I just couldn't face being so mean to myself anymore.

Something magical happened in those 30 days and in that mirror. The awful inner voice was replaced by a soft warm tone that emitted love and gratitude. It was very uncomfortable and hard but I did it for 30 days and I found I naturally made changes in other areas. I started to reduce consuming my trigger junk foods and my binge eating slowed down. I started to want to go to the gym. As I made these subtle changes, my body responded by slowly shrinking. My daily caressing of my wobbly bits started to instil pride at how it was changing. I was finally looking in the mirror with the "I am enough" phrase in my head and feeling like I could say it with pride, but I also knew I could and should do more.

Around this same time was when I started listening to David Goggins and heard his accountability mirror approach. Again, I did the same thing. I set myself a 30 day target and started to look in that mirror every night and ask "Did I give it my all today?" "Did I do my most valuable work today?" "What am I proud of today?" "What could I have done more of today?".

Asking yourself these questions while looking at your reflection does something to you from the inside out. Looking at yourself when you are not a vain person is difficult. When you've felt so uncomfortable in your own skin for so long and you no longer recognise the person staring back at you, it can be an emotional process. Yet slowly but surely I asked myself the difficult questions and gave myself the answers. Sometimes these mirror sessions then formed a journaling session, or the answers might pop up in a meditation. This process, like many of the others I mention in this book, were all interwoven.

The Accountability Mirror for an anti-procrastination quick fix

If you've just flicked to this chapter and you're looking for a quick fix and way out of procrastination then this is it.

Ideally you want to be able to do this where you can speak or shout out loud (I find sitting in my car for a minute is a good place to escape to, to complete this exercise and then get your ass into gear).

Take yourself off to the mirror. Set a timer for five minutes. It seems like a long time - that's because it is! For good reason.

Stare at your reflection for five minutes. Do nothing else. Fix your eyes on your gaze and just look at your own reflection.

Notice what comes up for you in your mind as you do this exercise. Think of it as conscious meditation. Your mind may whirr and wander. That is normal.

At the end of the five minutes, when the timer goes off, say to yourself aloud in the mirror what you are going to do right now. What action are you taking immediately after looking in the mirror and why is it important to you? Remind yourself that you are capable. Remind yourself of your talents and skills, your determination and drive. Make yourself a promise in the mirror there and then that you will take that first action step RIGHT NOW.

Look in the mirror, say "I am enough" out loud and go take action now.

Chapter 24

Audit Your Phone Use
(The Reassess, Realise and Re-Commit Process)

*

Affirmation: I appreciate that time is as valuable as money, thus I use every minute wisely.

Journal Prompt: Use the guidelines in this chapter and complete the reassess, realise and re-commit process for auditing your phone use.

*

My greatest problem is my mobile phone use. It could be social media, messaging friends and family on WhatsApp or using apps. I spent a lot of time on my phone and everyone around me noticed. I'd always lie and say I was catching up on emails but the truth was I was just wasting time and procrastinating on it - as usual!

I started off by deleting the Facebook app from my phone. I abstained from posting on Facebook, unless it was for clients, for three months. After that three month period, apart from sometimes being aware in conversations with friends and family that I'd missed certain photos or posts online, I realised we were communicating about anything important offline so I hadn't missed anything at all in those three months. I'd reclaimed a lot of time I'd usually be mindlessly scrolling.

Next I introduced charging my phone downstairs. Truth be told, in removing the Facebook app from my phone I just spent more time on Instagram and Twitter. It's like I'd replaced one vice with another. My phone use was the worst late at night in bed and also often resulted in me online shopping when I was half asleep. The packages from Amazon or eBay would turn up a few days later and I'd be genuinely surprised - forgetting I'd ordered them in the first place.

During this period where I was becoming more aware of my mobile phone use, we went on holiday to Turkey. When we landed I tried to connect to the Turkish mobile network. The data costs were astronomical. I worked out that my standard data use would cost me around £250 for the week if I were to agree to the Turkish network terms. I couldn't justify £250 to essentially spend a week on a beach scrolling through pictures of other people's lives, cat videos and the news. So my phone was turned off and placed in the safe and I was completely present for my whole family for the week.

Not having my phone by my face late at night also had a positive impact on my sleep quality. I was falling asleep naturally at 10pm every night and for the first time in years enjoying around 9-10 hours of amazing sleep each night. I felt recharged and renewed.

So when we returned home, I made a commitment that my phone would never be charged by my bed again. That was seven months ago as I write this chapter. It has had such a positive impact on my sleep, the quality of my sleep, my spending habits and my energy levels during the day.

The Reassess, Realise and Re-Commit Process

I find this hard to write because I too spend far too much time on my mobile phone and I'd go as far as to say I have a slight addiction. If you are in the Generation X, Y or Millennial category my bet is you too spend too much time on technology and it probably is one of your greatest sources of procrastination.

I don't want to look back on my life in my later years and have regrets of how I spent my time. I have to be strict with my phone use so that it doesn't cost me my job, my future books, my family time and my sleep.

So I came up with this process when chatting to teenagers about their mobile phone use in my speeches around discipline. I feel if you own a mobile phone or tablet then you too may benefit from looking into this process.

Reassess

First of all you can't be in denial when it comes to your mobile phone usage. You need to admit to yourself that you spend too much time on it and that starts with assessing where you are.

To do this, follow the reassess process:

- Go into your mobile phone settings.
- Hit 'screen time' and see what your daily average use is.
- Go into your activity breakdown and make a note of how long you spend on each of the apps.
- Do a weekly average and daily average. See what you spend your time on at the weekends compared to the weekdays.
- Notice at what times your use is high. Are there patterns?
- Tot up your top 5 apps and a weekly time spent on each.

Here are mine for this particular week:

YouTube 5 hr 41 mins

WhatsApp 4 hr 57 mins

Instagram 4h 25 mins

Facebook 4 hr 21 mins

UNRD 2h 38 mins

Total: 22 hours 3 minutes

Realise

This is the next step in the process and the one that is the most uncomfortable and difficult.

Look at your totals and make some realisations.

What is your weekly time spent on your phone?

What apps are taking most of your attention?

What is this time costing you?

That's almost a full day of my life, every week, on my phone.

As I am typing this out I feel disappointed. I have put so many measures in place to reduce my phone use and while those are weekly totals and the Facebook and Instagram usage has reduced considerably, it is still a long time to have my eyes and hands on my device.

WhatsApp is always a busy app for me, but being honest if I didn't message people first as much, I wouldn't be waiting for replies and then therefore spend more time on it. I could also probably call some of my friends and get the answers I need in one call rather than a few hours of back and forth messaging.

UNRD is a clever storytelling app. Instead of reading a book, this is a story played out through someone's mobile phone. The app is laid out like you have access to the protagonist's mobile phone and you can essentially read all their messages, watch all their live streams and be immersed in their world. The messages and notifications are delivered in real time and it's brilliant, but I now realise it is also slightly addictive and it is costing me too much time. I don't like it enough for it to take 2hrs and 38 minutes out of my week.

Realising what your apps cost you in time and understanding where and why you want to cut your use will help you on the next stage of this three part plan.

Re-Commit

It's time to re-commit to new phone habits now that you have reassessed your phone use and realised what this time is costing you.

At this stage, what can you commit to moving forwards?

Could you put restrictions on some apps you use too much?

How can you reduce the phone use and why is it important to you?

Remember - decreasing your phone use will give you valuable time back that you can use to work on your goals, practise meaningful relaxation or strengthen relationships.

Chapter 25

Factor in Some Play

Affirmation: I am cultivating joy and playfulness every day. Life is fun and full of wonderful surprises and magic.

Journal Prompt: Where can I factor in more playtime in my life? Which parts of my life are rather serious and could do with some light and laughter?

*

Playing around does not necessarily mean a lack of focus and effort. Sometimes if life is too serious and rigid this creates inner conflict which in turn can create procrastination.

We procrastinate on the stuff we don't want to do. The stuff that is dull and boring and serious. Now what you might deem fun might be dull to someone else and vice versa. For example, I hate spreadsheets. Always have and always will. My lack of experience and knowledge with Excel causes me to hate any task involving a spreadsheet. I have no confidence using it so if it is required that I use it for a presentation or budgeting or any aspect of formulas I will freak out and most certainly put that task off. In contrast, my friend Helen runs her business, Insight Finance Solutions, and as an accountancy adviser Helen is the MOST excitable and enthusiastic person when it comes to spreadsheets. She gets such a personal buzz and thrill compiling reports and spreadsheets because it is her zone of genius. We are all different in our approach and so we need to assess what is fun and light compared to what is a drain and heavy when it comes to our goals and tasks.

In Perspectives on Psychological Science, researchers Meredith Van Vleet and Brooke Feeney defined exactly what play in adults is and what it is not[1].

Van Vleet and Feeney define play as:

> *A behaviour or activity carried out with the goal of amusement and fun that involves an enthusiastic and in-the-moment attitude or approach, and is highly interactive among play partners or with the activity itself.*

When talking about play in the workplace, research has found evidence that play at work is often a positive. The modern day workforce actively commands play as part of their working lives. Think of big companies like Google and Facebook. Their modern office spaces are thriving with spaces and objects directly linked to play. Whether that be table tennis spaces, gaming stations, sporting spaces or chill out zones, these are all spaces within a working environment where you can break from the slog, play a while, ignite a little energy and creativity into your day and increase innovation.

Play at work has been linked to positive benefits including less fatigue, boredom, stress, and burnout in employees. Play and having the space to play and look at the lighter side of work helps increase job satisfaction, competence and creativity. There are numerous studies that have shown employees enjoy tasks and engage more when they are presented by their leaders in a playful way[2]. A study by Warwick University showed that happiness makes people more productive in work and experiencing joy through play in the workplace directly affected happiness and employee satisfaction levels[3].

When play is factored into a working team with employees from different levels coming together, it increases trust, bonding, social interaction, innovation, creativity, solidarity, loyalty and helps diffuse traditional hierarchies which often stifle great ideas and collaboration. When play is an active part of an organisation, data reveals that whole organisations benefit from a friendlier working atmosphere, more balance, higher employee commitment and productivity, more flexibility, better whole organisation decision making and ideas generation.

However there is an alternative and darker side to play at work. Forced play doesn't work[4]. Everyone has to consent and not everyone will feel comfortable playing - particularly if the order of play has not come from leaders. Play is also not as prominent in workforces with older employees[5]. You can't expect someone close to retirement who has worked one way their whole life to suddenly want to shoot a game of pool or have a go on the company Playstation in their lunch break. You should never enforce play on someone who is not comfortable participating.

Millennials will make up 75% of the workforce by 2025 and so play is not something that modern day employers can ignore. Rigid rules in a modern workplace do not necessarily work. Being human in the workplace is your superpower. There is a definite shift towards being more vulnerable and your true self at work to command more interaction, honesty and collaboration between team members.

While the above is food for thought for managers and those in leadership roles, if you're someone reading this who cannot fathom how play could possibly enter your working life, consider what you could do yourself as an individual. While you might not be able to change the whole culture of your organisation overnight, you do have the personal ability and responsibility to be able to change your own mood and therefore influence the happiness of those colleagues around you and yourself. When you are more satisfied in your work, you are more productive. A little bit of corporate play acts as a good break and can provide the right environment and time to feel more creative and therefore drive innovation. When you're in a state of innovation you are in 'flow' and therefore productive.

Chapter 26

The Dopamine Fast and Digital Detox

Affirmation: I remain focused on my important tasks. I do not succumb to distractions.

Journal Prompt: Where am I seeking instant gratification in my life? What can I not resist that always stops me feeling focused?

*

In 2019 'dopamine fasting' became a bit of a buzzword trend in Silicon Valley after a professor and dopamine faster, Dr. Cameron Sepah started to treat app developers and coding experts working at Silicon Valley's top digital companies for their overwhelm and lack of focus[1]. He uses the fasting as a technique in clinical practice with his clients as a way to reduce daily stimulation and reset the brain's sensory receptors.

Dopamine is the chemical that is associated with how we feel pleasure. It is a neurotransmitter, that when exchanged with other neurotransmitters in different parts of the brain, drives our behaviour. Dopamine helps control our response to rewards like food, sex and drugs so Dr Sepah determined that a rush of dopamine was to blame for destructive behaviours that would alter the pattern of productivity for the creative digital types he was treating in his clinical setting. Devotees of dopamine fasting can take it to the extreme and some would abstain from social media, internet, TV, food, sex and in some cases even eye contact and verbal communication with friends. The idea behind dopamine fasting is that abstaining from all forms of pleasure and stimulation will reset the brain's receptors and allow these people to become more focused, think more clearly and see themselves with more clarity.

While we do need dopamine for our brains to function, Dr Sepah advocates fasting from all pleasures and stimuli for as long as possible. Most devotees of dopamine fasting will practise this for a 24-48 hour period, usually over a weekend, with a goal to start work again on a Monday morning feeling revitalised and ready to focus.

Not all scientists agree and Dr Emiliano Merlo from the School of Psychology at the University of Sussex responded to the news of the rise in dopamine fasting saying; "I do not know any piece of scientific literature that will give empirical support for the explanation that the participants are giving for dopamine fasting.

"Perhaps these fasting periods are positive for many aspects, which makes them valid, but the idea that removing yourself from some particular behavioural activity reduces dopamine levels in the brain is extremely speculative. The so-called reboot effect might be more closely associated with reducing sensory saturation than any effects on the dopamine system."

I thought I'd include both sides of this argument in this book and allow you to make your own judgement whether you think this might work for you. Whether you call it a dopamine fast, delayed gratification or just abstaining from certain behaviours, there's power in having the discipline to say no or delaying things that bring us pleasure. A dopamine fast would see you abstain from food, any form of technology, exercise, touching your own or another person's body, music, raising your heart rate too much, communicating with others and heading outdoors to anywhere crowded. It would be up to you how long your own dopamine fast would last but would it be enlightening or incredibly boring?

The Vipassana silent meditation retreats that take place all over the world would act as a dopamine fast. Vipassana meditation commands non-reaction to your surroundings, thoughts or the pain as you sit still on a cold floor for hours with numb limbs and a brain aching for a break. While mindfulness meditation might focus on your awareness or transcendental meditation uses mantra, Vipassana encourages you to focus on the rise and fall of your body as you scan your limbs in a specific order. The idea is that by doing this for a 10 day period, you will reset your brain and stop yourself reacting so quickly to everyday events, thoughts, emotions and sensations. When you commit to a 10 day Vipassana practice you agree to abide by strict rules: no killing, no stealing, no lying, no sexual misconduct and no intoxicants. No writing, no talking, no eye contact and no communicating. You don't need to effectively put yourself in solitary confinement for 10 days to 'reset' your brain. Sometimes all you need to do is reset your worst habits and for many of us, that means taking an extended break from your digital life.

Try a digital detox

When was the last time you went on vacation? When you go on vacation do you sit by the pool with your mobile phone in hand for the duration of your stay? When we go on holiday, mobile technology makes it easy to stay connected but that also means we stay connected to our jobs, never really taking that well-needed break. We go on holiday to rest and relax but we check our emails, respond to our colleagues and scroll social media. Apps like WhatsApp mean we've got work group chats in our private messaging inbox and unless we take a break from these too, are we actually getting a chance to recharge our batteries, lower our cortisol levels and return from our holidays feeling refreshed?

The same can be said for our home lives. Once we have clocked off from our jobs, many of us are still connected to our work and our colleagues through our email and messaging apps. You might have the Slack app buzzing away late into the evening, or your emails pinging late at night and early in the morning - you can't seem to escape. Even reading endless and constant streams of news updates can leave you feeling overwhelmed and anxious.

This is where a digital detox comes in. It doesn't have to be as drastic as a 10 day silent meditation retreat and it doesn't mean you have you fast from your whole life for 24 hours. If you have been stuck on a task that you really want to complete or you want to adopt some positive productivity habits into your life then having a digital detox on a regular basis could really help you.

I talked in Chapter 24 about my own phone use. I have always spent a lot of time on my phone and everyone around me notices. In the past, I'd always lie and say I was catching up on emails but the truth was I was often just mindlessly scrolling, looking for that next dopamine hit.

When trying to complete this book, I did another form of digital detox by reducing my TV watching time. I knew I needed to work hard to finish the edits of this book and get it ready to be published but I found the temptation of the latest must-see Netflix show once again acting as the ultimate time vacuum. This trashy reality show about people dating through a frosted window and then marrying a month later had me hooked. I was using the show as a reward after extended periods of hard work but found myself slipping so easily into watching the next episode and the next. I knew this was causing me more stress as the deadline to get the book draft completed passed. I asked my husband for help. I didn't want to admit that I was succumbing to procrastination again (while finishing a book on procrastination - the irony!) but I was brave and honest, asking him to help me stop binge watching the show. He did one simple thing for me - he logged me out of the Netflix account on all the TVs and devices we own. He knew I didn't know the password and knew this would stop me being able to consume any more shows. Bingo! It worked. I detoxed from Netflix for a week while I finished the book and used the rest of the trashy reality show as the final reward that would be mine once I'd completed my manuscript and sent it off for publishing.

Go greyscale

Remove the allure of notifications by taking the colour out of your phone screen when you're trying to focus. You have the ability to put your phone into greyscale mode through your phone settings which will mean all those red notifications turn to grey and those apps you're addicted to will no longer be bright, shiny, colourful and attractive to the eye.

To activate greyscale on an iPhone go to general > accessibility > display and text size > colour filters.

On Android the greyscale option is part of a suite of digital well-being tools. To activate this on Android go to quick settings panel > tap pen icon on lower left > drag greyscale icon up into the panel of icons. This will then give you a one-tap access to the greyscale mode on your phone whenever you need it.

Distraction apps

If you can't manage a full digital detox over an extended period of time, how about using distraction apps to reduce your phone use while you're trying to focus? At the time of going to print the following apps were popular for helping us curb our social media and internet use and get on with our work;

Self Control
This app is unfortunately only available for macs. You can set the app up to restrict access to social media, email or the whole of the internet. What I love about this app is that even if you turn off your computer and restart it, the app remembers the time limits you set and

won't override them! You can put stops on your distractions for up to 24 hours. This is a particularly good choice if you have children and teenagers who spend too much time on their devices.

Freedom
A little like Self Control but available on Mac, PC and Android, Freedom will clock the internet for up to 8 hours. This is good if you need your computer for focused work like writing a paper or dissertation, or even writing a book. Unlike Self Control you can reboot your computer and access the internet again.

Anti-Social
This is pretty good if you still need internet access to research but you don't want to access social media. Made by the same people who brought us Freedom, Anti-Social lets you block social media and other sites like Wikipedia for any time between 15 minutes and 8 hours.

LeechBlock
This is a Firefox add-on where you can set rules for accessing certain sites. For example you can set it to be able to access Twitter from 9am to 5pm on weekdays or let you look at Facebook for 10 minutes each hour.

StayFocused
StayFocused is a Chrome plugin a little like LeechBlock but instead of restricting access to sites, you can set time limits for use instead. For example, you might allocate an hour a day to Facebook. Once you have used up that time, you won't be able to access Facebook until the next day. It's like the reversal of restriction but leaves you in control of your usage.

FocusON
This is an app made for Android devices. You can choose to block access to sites or apps that you use too much using the app. You can schedule a timer to block things for a certain amount of time or set it to restrict access to apps and sites at set times each day.

Focus
Made specifically for Mac, this app blocks social networks and instant messaging over a certain period of time. It shows up in the menu bar next to the clock so even if you attempt to use different browsers it will put a stop to it. Focus also has an option like SelfControl where you can't override the settings - even if you quit the app.

Breaking from our digital lives, whether on a holiday or consciously at home or work while we try to focus, is always a good thing. You realise what you miss out on, you realise how much technology disconnects us when we are present with each other and you realise the cost of your dreams when you work out the time you waste on technology.

Chapter 27

Enjoy The Discomfort

Affirmation: I love to feel discomfort as I work towards my goals. Every difficult step gets easier.

Journal Prompt: Think back to a time when achieving a goal took you through a period of discomfort. How did you get through it? What areas of your life are difficult and full of discomfort but rewarding once achieved?

*

I talked about David Goggins in the Accountability Mirror chapter and I'm going to talk about him again in this chapter about learning to enjoy the discomfort. I mentioned in the mirror work chapter about listening to David's audiobook and podcast in one. It is 15 hours long so I listened on many dog walks late at night.

One night David is describing this race in Hawaii where he's attempting to run 130 miles in a 72 hour period. I was immersed in this story and many of the others he tells in that audio book and autobiography about his various endurance experiences. In this race he's describing running without a torch up and down treacherous hills, smelling the stench of nearby pigs and feeling his toe blisters pop. It's a gruelling listen and read. He tells this story through the book and subsequent audiobook discussion and it's so evident how much he loves doing this kind of thing. He talks about needing to 'callous the mind' and you can hear it in his voice how much of a kick he gets from seeing what he is capable of and how he can push his own mindset to beyond usual human mental limits.

It was really late this one night while I was out walking in the dark in the depths of winter. What David was describing during his Hawaii Hell Race was pretty much what I could see ahead of me too - pure pitch black, slippery surfaces, mud and my own stinking animals (my two dogs) close by. I was in my stiff walking boots and jeans, two jumpers, my long overcoat, head torch, gloves and scarf. I found myself feeling my heart rate rising as I listened to David recall every detail of this race. I was getting stirred up and excited! Out of nowhere I started to quicken my pace. Like you would in a gym class when that extra fast beat tune comes on. I couldn't help myself. Before I knew it, I was running. At speed. In jeans and walking boots with my dogs pulling like Husky dogs across the North Pole as we navigated the icy conditions. I ran a 3 mile loop that night while listening to David. In my jeans, layers, wireless headphones, head torch and boots. My heart rate peaked at 190bpm and I thought I might have a heart attack but as I got home I didn't want to slump on the floor or down a litre of water. I was pumped, psyched and I wanted to go again. My husband looked at me like I'd actually lost the plot. This poor man has been the sole witness to my previous breakdowns and I think he thought this time I'd gone the other way and psychosis with hysteria had set in.

I couldn't help myself. I was elated. I carried on listening to the audiobook as I towelled down the dogs, washed my walking boots and peeled off my sweat soaked clothes.

"You have to learn to enjoy the discomfort" David growled in his trademark no-nonsense, no-shit hard Navy SEAL voice.

It stopped me in my tracks. "Enjoy the discomfort? Enjoy?" I remember thinking to myself. David was right. If I'd set out that night with the conscious intention to run in my inappropriate clothing and footwear you can guarantee I probably would not have enjoyed it. Listening to David Goggins and being so in the moment, so motivated and so moved to run had seen my brain change from a state of unenthusiastic energy to euphoria. I *enjoyed* it. Which meant it had felt a lot easier to me.

I started to put this into practice in other areas. At a Monday morning circuit class run by the funniest, loudest and most energetic instructor Claire, I decided this week I'd join in with her singing and silly dance moves between exercises. Claire was famous for this, week in, week out. She did it to take our minds off the burpees, wall sits with a 20kg weight on your lap or the horrific assault bike intervals. I'd always loved her classes for her fun and infectious energy but thinking back, I did shirk off 5 seconds before the end of each exercise round. I did go on my knees during the press ups. I did pick up the lighter weight options on the deadlifts. I did all of this with a grimace and a mental countdown every time I glanced at my watch. I'd spent years counting down the minutes and seconds until the class was over and I could get out of there. This time I decided to reverse that. Thanks to the motivation of David Goggins. I made a conscious decision that I was going to enjoy the discomfort and I'd find ways of distracting myself from the muscle fatigue.

It was like a new me had taken over my body. The class was so much easier, more enjoyable and boy did I work extra hard! I sang my way through that class, danced with Claire on what should've been the rest periods and laughed so hard I swear the next day my abdominal muscles were crying.

I've used this same idea of enjoying discomfort when helping a colleague overcome her fear of public speaking. We created a series of mantras and affirmations around changing fear into enjoyment.

'I am growing professionally and personally every time I speak out loud.'

'I enjoy the feeling of discomfort when I speak aloud. It means I am getting out of my comfort zone and conquering my fears.'

'Every time I feel fearful on stage, I need to remember that nerves are good. Discomfort means I don't come across too cocky.'

'When I experience discomfort on stage, I smile inside knowing that I am finding new ways to adapt and change.'

Enjoying discomfort will allow you to push past the feeling of your lungs burning, your armpits chafing and your feet blistering as you aim for your sub 2 hour time on your next half marathon.

Enjoying discomfort will allow you to go for that promotion at work and stand up confidently to present your winning idea to your peers in your interview.

Enjoying the discomfort will allow you to live in a building site while you work on renovating your house.

Enjoying the discomfort will allow you to smile through every deadlift and bootcamp session as you burn body fat and change your physique.

Learning to switch actions that are uncomfortable or painful to feeling like important, exciting and enjoyable steps on a huge journey will make such a difference when you aim for your goals. Doing anything from a place of negativity will never feel good but you have the capability to change how you feel about a situation and view it with excitement and happiness, rather than loathing and dread. This doesn't take away the fear, the physical pain or the nerves but it allows you the opportunity to make a decision whether that discomfort is going to be something you cry about or smile about.

Chapter 28

Final Words

Procrastination is not all bad. Sometimes when we procrastinate our bodies and brains are showing us that we don't want to do something so procrastinating on tasks over and over again presents an opportunity to examine how you feel about this particular work in your life. Is it making you happy? Is it fulfilling your dreams and desires?

If it's the boring adult stuff like household chores that you procrastinate on and you're not in a position to hire in some help to lighten the load, then you have to find the joy in it. Learn to combine it with things you do love like maybe music or podcasts or dancing.

If you're procrastinating on any aspect of your outer appearance like trying to lose body fat, get fit or train for a sporting event then your tendency to procrastinate might be rooted in your fear of the overwhelming task ahead. When the overwhelm strikes, refer back to the chapters on setting that first step in two minutes or less. "I will run 30 miles every week" becomes "I will lace up my trainers three times a week". Start small and see where the action takes you.

If it is writing a book or setting up a business, our procrastination often comes from our fear of being visible and judged. What will people say? What if they hate it? We worry about this judgement, even on a subconscious level and it causes us to feel stuck and unable to take action.

When it comes to tasks in your work or your job in general, if you're muddling through every day and not performing at your best, which in turn is causing stress, then you get to have an opportunity to assess your career choice and firstly change your mindset around your work (trialling some of the anti-procrastination methods detailed in this book may help you feel more capable and confident at work before you decide to quit and find something else!). If you find that you improve your productivity at work and you're still not happy and still struggling to get over the procrastination, are you challenged enough? Could you aim for that promotion or retrain within the business to get on the next step of the career ladder? If not and you're still procrastinating you get to take responsibility and ask if it is time to find something else that will fulfil you. We spend such a lot of our adult lives in our jobs and we don't need to live for our vacations when there is so much rewarding and fulfilling work in the world.

Ultimately getting over procrastination is realising what you can control and what you can't. It is about trialling ways that will help you get out of your own way to then make you trust in your abilities. When you trust yourself, you believe in yourself and when you believe in yourself you know you're able to keep your promises to yourself and do the things that need to be done in order to have a happy and successful life.

I wish you the very best as you move forward in your own life. I hope the research, tips and anecdotal stories have helped inspire you to at least trial a few of the methods as explored in the book. I know my whole life has changed since I made a conscious decision to see what I was capable of in my life and business. I want that for you too.

In addition to my books I run a free Facebook group where members and I support each other through all aspects of productivity, self-discipline, happiness and having a great life. It is a place for those who love to do the work on themselves and drop the excuses to see what they can achieve.

If you have been inspired to take action after reading this book, I would love to hear about your story and journey. Please get in touch with me via my website at **www.gemmaray.com**

Here's to *you* achieving all your dreams and goals. Good luck!

Gifts from Me to You

As a thank you for downloading this book I would like to give you a couple of free gifts that I know will complement and strengthen the strategies outlined in this book.

Free Goal Setting Masterclass
This powerful session will help you get clear on your goals. When you know what you are aiming for and the meaningful reasons why, it gives you clarity.

Free Goal Setting Masterclass Workbook
It's easy to watch a masterclass about productivity but harder to implement the strategies, so follow the plan and the workbook.

Claim your free gifts at **www.gemmaray.com/bonus**

Acknowledgements

This book would not be possible without the unwavering support of my business partner, Ben Jones, who continues to crack the whip, tag me endlessly on Asana tasks and keep me in check. Ben is the antidote to my imposter syndrome which often keeps me stumped and overwhelmed. Thank you for your four glorious years of accountability, support, research, expertise and friendship.

Thank you to the members of our Facebook support group who have allowed me to mentor them on a journey overcoming procrastination. A special mention to Sarah Humphreys who continues to thrive on all the tips and loves accountability as much as I do.

Lots of love to my friend and mentor Laura Powner. You have been there for me in all the dark and all the light and I can't wait for our next cottage working retreat to help you write your own book.

Thank you Stacey and Michelle my SNDYVG ladies who are always only a WhatsApp message, or if we're lucky a Michelle-special voice note away. Your wisdom, laughter and advice is something I hold so dear to my heart.

My beta readers and proof readers including the grammar ninja Jenny Chalmers, the eagle eyed Polly Burns plus Karen Dequatre Cheeseman and Tiffany Huber whose eyes and comments were so helpful in ensuring this book read OK for a European, Australasian and American market. I shake my fist at autocorrect and fat fingers but your input and comments weeded out the mistakes and typos. I am so grateful to you for your help.

To Cate Butler-Ross who probably got very frustrated with my lack of writing progress during our mastermind but whose expertise has helped enormously and Jess Evans, thank you for passing on your knowledge to me too and being so encouraging and enthusiastic.

To Laura Hughes who believes in me more than I believe in myself at times. I just adore you and your energy always gives me a boost I need.

To my colleagues at the BBC, especially Nicola Adam, my work wife and co-host; thank you for your support and helping me seek out further opportunities to showcase my work.

To my husband Shaun and my son Blake, I am sorry I often kick you out of the house when it is time to write and I apologise for my crazy lightning speed typing that keeps you awake at night. I am doing this for you to hopefully create a life of a little more freedom to ensure we cultivate as many precious memories as possible.

Finally, to you my reader! Thank you for downloading this book and supporting a self-published author like myself. Please don't forget to leave a review when you have finished the book as it really helps support us 'Indies' (independent authors). You can get exclusive access to new book releases, free downloads, programme announcements and additional resources by signing up to the mailing list at **www.gemmaray.com**. I also publish a super helpful newsletter exclusively to my mailing list.

Appendix

Introduction

¹ The podcast that explains the rules and thought process behind #75Hard is outlined by creator Andy Frisella here - https://andyfrisella.com/blogs/mfceo-project-podcast/75hard-a-75-day-tactical-guide-to-winning-the-war-with-yourself-with-andy-frisella-mfceo291

² The 100 books on discipline list was published on the #75 Hard Dominators group on Facebook - https://www.facebook.com/groups/344934989529753/

Chapter 1

¹ Work and Days by Hesiod - https://en.wikipedia.org/wiki/Works_and_Days

² The Canterbury Tales - https://en.wikipedia.org/wiki/The_Canterbury_Tales

³ More information about Chaucer's ambitions for his Canterbury tales are outlined on the British Library website - https://www.bl.uk/collection-items/the-canterbury-tales-by-geoffrey-chaucer

⁴ It had been believed to have been painted between 1503 and 1506; however, Leonardo may have continued working on it as late as 1517 - https://en.wikipedia.org/wiki/Mona_Lisa

⁵ For further analysis and reading - https://opentextbc.ca/introductiontopsychology/chap-

ter/12-1-psychological-disorder-what-makes-a-behavior-abnormal/

[6] From the Cost of Interrupted Work: More Speed and Stress study by the University of California, Irvine - https://www.ics.uci.edu/~gmark/chi08-mark.pdf

[7] From Freud's Pleasure Principle - https://en.wikipedia.org/wiki/Pleasure_principle_(psychology)

[8] Darren Tong's article in full - https://alphaefficiency.com/4-types-procrastination-beat/

Chapter 2

[1] Hewitt and Flett's 45-item Multidimensional Perfectionism Scale - https://www.researchgate.net/publication/304344471_Comparing_Two_Short_Forms_of_the_Hewitt-Flett_Multidimensional_Perfectionism_Scale

[2] Positive Perfectionism: Seeking the Healthy "Should", or Should We? - https://pdfs.semanticscholar.org/20da/6cb1d6fc4cadc5c57a9736dbf5742087e61a.pdf

[3] Positive and negative perfectionism and their relationship with anxiety and depression in Iranian school students - https://www.ncbi.nlm.nih.gov/pmc/articles/PMC3063422/

[4] Riley et al 2007 Perfectionism: A randomised controlled trial of cognitive-behaviour therapy for clinical perfectionism: A preliminary study - https://www.ncbi.nlm.nih.gov/pmc/articles/PMC2777249/

Chapter 3

[1] The Five Second Rule by Mel Robbins - https://www.amazon.com/dp/B01MUSNFOO
[2] Descartes' Error: Emotion, Reason and the Human Brain - https://www.amazon.co.uk/dp/B0031RS9I4/

Chapter 4

[1] Self Discipline: A How-to Guide to Stop Procrastination and Achieve Your Goals in 10 Steps - www.mybook.to/selfdiscipline

² Getting Things Done: The Art of Stress Free Productivity - https://www.amazon.com/dp/B00SHL3V8M

Chapter 5

¹ Mike Vardy: Why Two-Minute Tasks Don't Work - https://productivityist.com/two-minute-warning

Chapter 6

¹ Implementation Intentions and Goal Achievement: A Meta-Analysis of Effects and Processes by Peter M. Gollwitzer and Pascal Sheeran - https://www.researchgate.net/publication/37367696_Implementation_Intentions_and_Goal_Achievement_A_Meta-Analysis_of_Effects_and_Processes

Chapter 8

¹ The Pomodoro Technqiue official website - https://francescocirillo.com/pages/pomodoro-technique

Chapter 9

¹ Bridging the information worker productivity gap - https://warekennis.nl/wp-content/uploads/2013/11/bridging-the-information-worker-productivity-gap.pdf

² Marie Kondo: The Life Changing Magic of Tidying Up - https://www.amazon.com/dp/B00I0C46BO/

³ The Organised Mum Method - https://www.theorganisedmum.blog/

Chapter 10

¹ Attenuating Neural Threat Expression with Imagination by Marianne Cumella Reddan, Tor Dessart Wager, and Daniela Schiller in Neuron. Published December 6 2018. Doi: 10.1016/j.neuron.2018.10.047

² They Did You Can by Michael Finnigan - https://www.amazon.com/dp/B008CPIY9Y

Chapter 11

[1] Flow: The Psychology of Optimal Experience by Mihaly Csikszentmihalyi - https://www.amazon.com/Flow-Psychology-Experience-Perennial-Classics/dp/0061339202

[2] Maslow's hierarchy of needs - https://en.wikipedia.org/wiki/Maslow%27s_hierarchy_of_needs

[3] The Transient Hypofrontality Theory of Altered States of Consciousness - https://www.researchgate.net/publication/333077072_The_Transient_Hypofrontality_Theory_of_Altered_States_of_Consciousness

[4] Flow: Instead of Losing Yourself, You are Being Yourself, Scott Barry Kauffman - https://scottbarrykaufman.com/flow-instead-of-losing-yourself-you-are-being-yourself/

Chapter 12

[1] "Around 40 percent of the population are morning people, 30 percent are evening people, and the reminder lies in between. Night owls aren't owls by choice. They are bound to a delayed schedule by unavoidable DNA hard wiring. It's not their conscious fault, but rather their genetic fate." - Dr Matthew Walker, Why We Sleep

[2] The Miracle Morning by Hal Elrod - https://www.amazon.com/dp/B013PKZUOW

Chapter 13

[1] I Forgive Myself, Now I Can Study - https://www.academia.edu/28728632/I_forgive_myself_now_I_can_study_How_self-forgiveness_for_procrastinating_can_reduce_future_procrastination

2 Dark Side of the Light Chasers - https://www.amazon.com/dp/1594485259

Chapter 14

[1] Everything is Figureoutable by Marie Forleo - https://www.amazon.co.uk/dp/B07N4DLLGS

Chapter 16

[1] You Need an Innovation Strategy, Harvard Business Review - https://hbr.org/2015/06/you-need-an-innovation-strategy

Chapter 18

[1] The 'Mozart Effect' study by Gordon Shaw, Frances Rauscher and Katherine Ky - https://www.ncbi.nlm.nih.gov/pmc/articles/PMC1281386/

[2] The Cardiovascular Effect of Musical Genres - A randomized controlled study on the effect of compositions by W. A. Mozart, J. Strauss, and ABBA - https://www.aerzteblatt.de/int/archive/article/179298/The-cardiovascular-effect-of-musical-genres-a-randomized-controlled-study-on-the-effect-of-compositions-by-W-A-Mozart-J-Strauss-and-ABBA

[3] Tuning the cognitive environment: Sound masking with "natural" sounds in open-plan offices - https://asa.scitation.org/doi/abs/10.1121/1.4920363

Chapter 19

[1] Intracranial electroencephalography power and phase synchronization changes during monaural and binaural beat stimulation - https://www.ncbi.nlm.nih.gov/pubmed/25345689#

Chapter 20

[1] Benefits of napping in healthy adults: impact of nap length, time of day, age, and experience with napping - https://onlinelibrary.wiley.com/doi/full/10.1111/j.1365-2869.2008.00718.x

[2] Take a Nap! Change Your Life.: The Scientific Plan to Make You Smarter, Healthier, More Productive - https://www.amazon.com/dp/B00B8UDC1U

[3] Andrew Johnson hypnotherapy apps - https://andrewjohnson.co.uk

Chapter 21

[1] Caffeine effects on sleep taken 0, 3, or 6 hours before going to bed - https://www.ncbi.nlm.nih.gov/pubmed/24235903

Chapter 22

[1] Weight loss social support in 140 characters or less: use of an online social network in a remotely delivered weight loss intervention - http://dx.doi.org/10.1007/s13142-012-0183-y

[2] Gretchen Rubin, Better Than Before - https://www.amazon.com/dp/B00PQJHIXM

[3] Willpower: Rediscovering the Greatest Human Strength Roy T. Baumeister and John Tierney - https://www.amazon.com/dp/B005TIVK7A

[4] American Society of Training and Development accountability study - https://books.google.co.uk/books?hl=en&lr=&id=mHTEkvyjaLwC&oi=fnd&pg=PR1&dq=astd+study+on+accountability&ots=Tl_zG176Yi&sig=qGr1ndwsihxE_Pd2ko0WhPtsuJk&redir_esc=y#v=onepage&q=astd%20study%20on%20accountability&f=false

[5] Goals Research Summary - https://www.dominican.edu/sites/default/files/2020-02/gailmatthews-harvard-goals-researchsummary.pdf as published here initially by Dr Gail Matthews - https://www.dominican.edu/directory-people/gail-matthews

Chapter 23

[1] Can't Hurt Me by David Goggins on Audible - https://www.audible.com/pd/Cant-Hurt-Me-Audiobook/B07KKMNZCH

[2] I Am Enough: Mark Your Mirror And Change Your Life by Marisa Peer - https://www.amazon.com/dp/B07HJBW7VB

Chapter 25

[1] Young at Heart: A Perspective for Advancing Research on Play in Adulthood by Meredith Van Vleet and Brooke C Feeney - https://journals.sagepub.com/doi/abs/10.1177/1745691615596789

[2] Games Managers Play: Play as a Form of Leadership Development by Ronit Kark - https://www.jstor.org/stable/41318071?seq=1

[3] Happiness and Productivity by Andrew J. Oswald, Eugenio Proto and Daniel Sgroi - https://

wrap.warwick.ac.uk/63228/7/WRAP_Oswald_681096.pdf

[4] The 'gamification of work processes is an "imposition" of managers on employees - https://books.google.co.uk/books?id=us-eBQAAQBAJ&lpg=PA155&dq=fleming%20and%20sturdy%202010%20mandatory%20fun&pg=PA155#v=onepage&q=fleming%20and%20sturdy%202010%20mandatory%20fun&f=false

[5] Play at Work: An Integrative Review and Agenda for Future Research - https://www.researchgate.net/publication/320047939_Play_at_Work_An_Integrative_Review_and_Agenda_for_Future_Research

Chapter 26

[1] Dopamine fasting: Misunderstanding science spawns a maladaptive fad - https://www.health.harvard.edu/blog/dopamine-fasting-misunderstanding-science-spawns-a-maladaptive-fad-2020022618917

Made in the USA
Coppell, TX
28 October 2021